Sanity and Strength:

Wisdom to Get Unstuck and
Power to Move on from the
Muddy Paths of Life Transitions

TOLU ADELEYE, PhD

Dedication

To those who having experienced loss or major changes in their circumstances are seeking to discover new purpose for their lives or career.

Table of Contents

INTRODUCTION

Sometimes life seems easy. The sky is clear and it feels like everything you want is possible. During these enjoyable periods you feel like you are heading down a smooth, easy-to-travel path of predictable day-to-day routines. But then, all of a sudden, you experience change and you are thrust off of the nice, smooth path onto one that is muddy, slippery, and filled with potholes. At first you are shocked and confused, because there was no warning that your path was going to change and you were totally unprepared as a result. But there you are in the middle of the muddy track. You try to pull out quickly, but find yourself sinking deeper into the slippery muck.

Slippery, Muddy Tracks

Life transitions are in many ways similar to that slippery, muddy track. One day you are well employed with great career prospects, the next day you have no job. One month you are happily married and raising your kids with a bright future, the next month your spouse serves you with divorce papers. One year you and your family are well established in a nice neighborhood in your city with what seems like unstoppable personal growth ahead. The next year your city is invaded by a hurricane and all that you have built over a significant part of your life gets washed away in an instant.

Just like being trapped on a slippery, muddy path, life transitions can be nerve-wracking. Initially they tend to leave you in a state of inertia, where you have no motivation even to move. Figuring out how to get unstuck requires wisdom and emotional strength on your part—resources that may not be very easy to access at such times. You may feel like you are going through the right motions but getting nowhere. The many attempts you make to get yourself unstuck may leave you sapped of all your energy.

When you finally are able to get unstuck, you may want to remain in what seems like a safe position. However, staying glued to one spot will not help you reach your originally desired destination. You will need even more wisdom to redesign your itinerary and find a new path to follow. In addition, you need a new inflow of strength to continue your journey and reach your desired goal in your new circumstances.

Wisdom and Strength to Navigate through Difficult Changes

Just having to go through a single life-changing event is challenging enough for any individual. Having to go through more than one earth-shattering change in quick succession places an enormous demand on even emotionally strong people.

Take Samantha. After graduating from college in the town where she had grown up, she secured a promising position with a firm in a different city. Although she is grateful for employment, she is a bit stressed about having to leave the security of a familiar environment and tackle the issues associated with an unfamiliar one.

Samantha gradually settles into her new position, and before she knows it, her six-month employment probation period is over. But just as she is starting to feel more settled again, Samantha learns that her mom has passed away. She is devastated at the news. Then, a few weeks after her mom's funeral, Samantha's fiancé breaks up with her. Samantha feels like curveballs are being thrown at her from every angle. How is she supposed to absorb all the changes in her life? How can she find the sanity to stay on top of all of them?

She decides to take some time off work to sort herself out. But as the end of her leave draws near, she finds it hard to summon the energy to go back to her employment. How and where is she going to find the strength to move on?

Samantha's feelings of being overwhelmed are understandable. We experience stressors of various kinds in our day-to-day lives, but during periods of transition, stress escalates. Stress takes a high toll on an individual, so anything that exposes someone to high amounts of prolonged stress is intimidating. When periods of seeming insanity interrupt people's lives, it takes a significant amount of strength to gather momentum even after the stress is removed or reduced.

Let me share another example. Danny started his career as a professional basketball player at a young age. He also invested in several promising business ventures early in his professional life. He really enjoys his career, and his personal life is going well too. He and his wife have a young son who means the entire world to them.

One day, Danny's journey on a smooth, paved road is diverted onto a muddy track when his son is diagnosed with a rare form of muscular dystrophy. Danny and his wife spend a lot of effort getting him the best treatments, traveling often over a long period of time to give him the care he needs. However, he does not seem to be responding well to the treatments.

Danny is hit with another blow when he finds out that his wife had been cheating on him. He wants to try and resolve the issues with her, but the concurrent health problems of his son have sapped a lot of his emotional strength. Danny seems to lack motivation, and sometimes he feels weak at the thought of starting fresh on a new path to rebuild his marriage. Where is he supposed to get new strength to carry on?

Both Samantha and Danny require enormous amounts of wisdom and strength to navigate through their complex transitions. If, like them, you are facing upheaval in your life, you also need these things so you can get through the difficult period and come out on top. *Sanity and Strength* will show you how to do just that.

Sanity and Strength: A Powerful Duo!

Sanity and strength are an inseparable pair on the pathway of a transition. It could be that you have experienced a breakup of a significant relationship, such as in divorce or the dissolution of a business. You might have lost something of great significance, such as a job or a career. Or maybe your loss is that of a lifestyle pattern, such as in retirement or relocation. Perhaps you experienced the loss of a spouse or a family member. Or you may be a survivor of a natural disaster such as a hurricane, in which almost everything you had was wiped away. All of these scenarios have a huge impact on you as a person. To find your way through the complexities of any of these transitions or similar ones, you need to acquire the duo of sanity and strength. The process to do so, both to mobilize yourself out of the inertia caused by the change and move on thereafter, is the subject of this book.

Sanity and strength are required both individually and in combination to manage a life transition successfully. They are needed even more to tackle the complexities of multiple life transitions that occur simultaneously. Both sanity and strength are needed at all stages of a change as you unravel the intricacies of the period, walk your way through it, and move on with your life thereafter.

Specifically, sanity is required to:

- Stay on top of the transition(s) and not be overwhelmed
- Downgrade the negative reactions to the emotional crisis that hits you and makes you feel helpless about your new situation
- Maintain a level of positivity to help you see light at the end of the tunnel
- Keep an open mind about exciting possibilities in the future

- Clarify where you want to go next and make the right choices for your new circumstances
- Decipher how to get to your newly desired position

Strength is required to:

Stay emotionally on top of your circumstances, especially at the beginning of the change when confusion saps your energy

- Cope with all the physical and emotional challenges posed by the change
- Do all that is required to get unstuck, such as shifting gears and getting rid of factors that are holding you down in the muddy path
- Move on with your journey when you finally get unstuck
- Take the actions required to get you to a new position

Sanity and strength are required in combination to:

- Counter any negative feedback or new obstructions you might face when you set out for your newly desired position
- Reinforce your identity in your new position
- Help you reach out to others with the same message of "wisdom to get unstuck and power to move on"
- Grasp opportunities to multiply your success by giving back to your community

In tandem, sanity and strength will go a long way to ease the stresses associated with life transitions. Sanity and strength will open the door to all that it takes for you to not only come out on the other side of change, but achieve more success on your new path. However, sanity and strength are not items you can buy off the shelf at a given price. They can be acquired only through your active input into the transition journey, and you need to know what kind of input is required and how you can offer this input during the navigation process.

This book addresses the subject of how you can acquire sanity and strength all along your journey of change. It provides you with proven strategies and practical tips to obtain the wisdom and strength to get unstuck, redesign your path, and subsequently move along this new path with success.

What's in This Book for You

In Chapter 1 you will learn how periods of stability are like walking on smooth, paved roads, and how you can use such periods to become change-ready. Chapters 2 to 8 then examine the period when that smooth, paved road turns into the muddy path of a life transition. In these seven chapters I have employed a framework of seven powerful questions that will evoke discovery, create self-awareness, and elicit action at various phases of your change.

Chapters 2, 3, and 4 discuss the stuck phase—the period just after you encounter the change. In Chapter 2 you will learn how to get the confusion out about the transition you just experienced. It describes how to acknowledge that your situation has changed and identify which factors have changed in it. Chapter 3 takes on the closely linked topic of delineating what caused the change in your circumstances. It equips you to take stock, express your feelings about the cause of the change, and mourn your loss. In Chapter 4 you will find out how loss impacts your identity and how to come to terms with this reality.

Chapters 2 to 4 prepare you to take on the essential task of the next phase: getting unstuck. Chapter 5 examines this concept in detail. It explains how you can get rid of the sticky factors holding you down and preventing you from moving on. Among other things, you will learn how to get rid of your fears about the change.

After getting unstuck, you need to move on. Chapters 6, 7, and 8 examine this moving-on phase. In Chapter 6 you will discover how to decipher your new destination by analyzing your options and examining your life's purpose. Chapter 7 equips you with tools for getting to your new place of choice. Among other things, you will learn how to search for and embrace a new identity for your new journey. Chapter 8 explains the equally important task of stabilizing yourself on your new journey and ensuring that you make it through to a new you.

Chapter 9 provides insight on how you can impact your community by sharing the lessons you learned from your experience. It empowers you to take on dreams larger than you and thereby find even more meaning in life.

To explain the principles for moving through change, I have employed the imagery of a truck that is stuck in a muddy path. You will meet Brian, the driver of the truck, and see how he is able to get his stuck truck out of the track and continue his journey to his destination of choice. Drawing analogies from his situation to your own, you will glean useful insights on how to get unstuck and move on during your period of change.

Throughout the book you will also meet people just like you who are going through challenging life transitions—job loss, divorce, loss of a loved one, physical disability, natural disaster, and illness. You will see how they use principles illustrated in *Sanity and Strength* to navigate their way through change and lead meaningful lives thereafter.

Sanity and Strength will empower you to:

- Unravel the complexities of the change you have experienced
- Overcome the lethargy created by the change as you clarify issues and discover what needs to be resolved
- Seek, develop, and embrace a new identity for moving forward
- Set and work on goals for bridging the gap between where you are now and where you would like to be in the future
- Take ownership of your new status and achieve success in your new circumstances

In addition, the book will equip you with tools for impacting your community through sharing. All in all, Sanity and Strength will empower you to use your period of change as a stepping stone to greater fulfillment in life.

I now invite you to come with me on a journey toward obtaining the sanity and strength required to navigate any life transitions and career changes that come your way.

PHASE 1

BEFORE GETTING STUCK

BEFORE GETTING STUCK

Welcome to the stable phase of your life where day-to-day events follow fairly predictable patterns. Count it as a phase of rest in which normal growth is taking place. It is the phase between major life transitions, and it is where you, like the majority of people, likely desire to be most of the time. It is calm, pleasant, comfortable, and enjoyable, and there are minimal interruptions to your life.

However, as discussed in upcoming chapters, the stable phase where no transition exists also tends to be one of minimal growth or personal development. Too much comfort often leads to a lack of vigor for development.

I must reiterate that we need such stable stages from time to time in our lives. However, the reality is that this stage does not last forever. Life must continue and growth is necessary for meaningful life to progress.

Chapter 1 describes in depth what it means to be in that elusive phase of normality, and why you should use this period to prepare for the inevitability of change.

Chapter 1

THE ELUSIVE SMOOTH, PAVED ROAD

Roads of various structures and engineering have been of interest to me lately. I find it fascinating that there is such a wide variety of road structures. My curiosity has been especially piqued in terms of how a road's design is based on the potential use to which it will be put.

On Different Road Construction Styles

In the developed world, well-engineered road structures are often taken for granted by the residents. These high-quality roads are well maintained and have minimal obstructions on them. They are well marked with appropriate road signs so there are no ambiguities for the drivers traveling on them. These well-developed roads range from highways with multiple lanes that can accommodate many vehicles traveling at high speed, to single-lane, solidly constructed streets in residential areas where there is less traffic. Roads in commercial and industrial areas have solid construction styles that can support heavy trucks and delivery vehicles. In all these cases, the road styles and construction fit with the use to which these roads are put.

Road styles in developing countries are less fancy. While urban centers usually have good highways, rural areas do not always enjoy the presence of high-quality road infrastructure. Depending on the location, you may encounter different surprises on your journey. In rural areas roads can shift dramatically from paved, fairly smooth roads to those with minimal paving, and then to winding, untarred roads with potholes.

From Well-maintained Highways to Unpaved, Ambiguous Roads

There is a huge contrast between traveling on a well-paved, smooth road and an unpredictable, unpaved road.

Highways lend themselves to high speeds—in fact, the cruise control feature that allows drivers to set the speed of their vehicle at a certain level and automate a major aspect of driving is possible because of the smoothness and predictability of such roads.

However, no driver ever attempts to use cruise control on an untarred road! On the contrary, the driver journeying on untarred terrain has to be very alert and travel at a low speed to survive the drastic navigational changes encountered on such a surface. In fact, it is not just the longevity of the vehicle that is at stake. The manner of traveling on such roads also impacts the health of the driver. At too high a speed, the up and down vibrations and movements into and out of potholes will take a toll on even the strongest of human physiques.

If life were a road, the smooth, paved surface is the one on which you most likely desire to travel. It stretches before you during periods of stability and predictability in your life when you need only a little effort for maintenance. It represents periods when there are no unpredicted changes or rude interruptions to your life like those posed by life transitions. When your life is stable and your day-to-day activities can be predicted to a significant extent, you encounter less stress and can assert without reservation that life is generally good. You can even afford to set many of your day-to-day functions on autopilot—just like when using the cruise control function of the car.

But then, out of nowhere, "life happens." You lose something of importance that you worked on for a good number of years. Maybe the loss is that of a job or career, material wealth, status, a relationship, or vital health parameters, but whatever the case, that smooth, paved road you were traveling on at high speed turns dramatically into an untarred road with potholes and little predictability. The sudden change may have caught you unawares. Your speed drops dramatically and you might even hit a place of no motion at all.

The smooth, paved road of life tends to be elusive for significant periods of time. It is sometimes vague or abstract, and may even seem indescribable to you since it exists only for certain periods of time over which you have only minimal control. The real fact is that transitions are a natural part of life. For growth and progress to happen, you must experience transitions. To develop in significant ways you must occasionally be tossed from that smooth, paved road of cruise control to an unpredictable one where you might be brought to a standstill for a period of time.

Hitting a Standstill on an Untarred, Pothole-ridden Road

Periods of standstill are even more prolonged if you experience multiple transitions concurrently.

As a waitress in a local restaurant, Catherine works morning shifts to put herself through college. She attends evening courses and is a very diligent student. Everything seems to be going well; she is happy with her progress and is looking forward to completing her course within a year.

One morning at work, Catherine receives news that her father, who lives about a five-hour drive away, has had a stroke and has been taken to the hospital. Catherine leaves her city quickly to be with her dad, but unfortunately, he passes away before she arrives. She takes time off work and her studies to be with her family during this period of loss.

When she returns home, Catherine finds that her apartment has been affected by a fire that broke out on the same floor of her building. Although some of her items are still intact, a significant amount of her belongings have been destroyed.

While she is trying hard to make some meaning out of these events, Catherine receives yet another blow when she discovers that the application deadline has passed for the internship placement for her professional registration. This means she has to wait another full year before she can get her credential. Catherine feels like her smooth, paved road has disappeared altogether. With no period for recovery between transitions, Catherine's life journey during this period seems to be on an untarred road filled with numerous potholes.

Transitions Are a Natural Part of Our Lives

As described above, transitions are like detours from your smooth, paved road. But for life to continue, we must experience change. Transitions are a natural part of human progression. We experience natural transition events such as birth, marriage, parenthood, retirement, and grandparenthood. These are all normal processes that happen during the course of our lives. The fact is, life is defined by change and change gives birth to life. Humans are faced with the certainty of death and the richness of new life as we walk this world.

This natural progression of transition and growth is exemplified in other occurrences, such as the process of metamorphosis. Metamorphosis, a biological transformation process, signifies a complete or marked change in the form of an animal as it develops into an adult—for example, the change from tadpole to frog or from caterpillar to butterfly. Metamorphosis is an alteration in form as well as growth. In true metamorphosis, the subject changes while it is in the process of becoming. The caterpillar grows in a cocoon until it is too big to be contained by it, at which point it must be liberated from that contained space to become what it is supposed to be: a beautiful butterfly. In similar ways, natural processes of transition stir us up in our little nests of comfort and stimulate us to get up and become who we are meant to be.

Types of Transitions

In addition to transitions that are natural parts of human life (birth, marriage, empty nest, retirement, old age), there are other categories of changes. There are those changes that may not be what you would choose normally but nevertheless embark upon because you see them as options for better success or fulfillment in your life. Remarriage, some cases of divorce, intentional career changes, and cross-country or international relocations are examples of this type of change. Although you tend to know about this type of change beforehand, you still find it challenging to take on because it requires adaptability in many areas of your life.

Other changes are termed as catastrophic events: changes that happen suddenly and unexpectedly, such as the loss of a job, a sudden divorce, the death of a loved one, a life-threatening disease, or a natural disaster. These unanticipated changes throw you out of balance and often make you question, "Why me? Why now?" These unplanned-for changes are like transitioning from the smooth highways to the unpaved roads of life.

Emotional Crisis Periods Are Like Paved Roads Full of Bumps

Another category of change you may experience is linked to emotional crisis that makes you question existential issues. During certain periods of your life you might have this inner quest for meaning and purpose. This could happen for no apparent reason in midlife or at times when you have an itch for something more fulfilling than the condition in which you find yourself. At such times you may question, "Why am I here? Is my life significant? Am I worthy?"

Periods of emotional crisis can be due to changes in the identity of an individual who has experienced an earth-shattering transition. A middle-aged executive who lost his twin brother could not cope with the situation for a long time. He and this brother had always planned vital family functions together for both of their families. This included their kids' education, family holidays, and even real estate and other investments.

After his brother's death, it was very difficult for this middle-aged man to continue planning these vital life events all on his own. He wanted to continue to lead and be there for his own family, but he also felt highly responsible for his deceased brother's family. Over time, the effort of trying to carry on two identities at once created tension for him, and the situation had unwanted effects on his immediate family. His wife had to work extra hard to get his attention and they started to grow apart. She tried to help him see how they could manage the situation better and invited him to seek professional help, but he refused. Thus, in this executive's life, one life-changing event that was not managed well eventually led to a series of emotional crises that impacted his work and family life.

Emotional crises, whether at midlife or at other times, can lead to a series of reactions that can be dangerous or even disastrous. If not managed properly, emotional crises may lead to multiple life transition events. Thus, periods of emotional crisis are like paved roads full of bumps. Such roads are difficult to travel.

Change Is Constant

As explained above, constant change is all around us. Whether we like it or not, change regularly happens in our lives and in the lives of all those we cherish. But continuous change also helps us grow. This positive aspect of continuous change is well illustrated by the meeting point between two different bodies of water. On long stretches of beach are places where the fresh water of a river or stream pours into the salt water of the ocean. Such points of confluence where a river meets the sea are referred to as estuaries. As the tide rises, the salt water pushes its way back into the fresh water, and eventually this force creates a shallow tidal basin.

Estuaries are places of continuous change; they are in constant transition. They change with the seasons, the tides, the wind, and the rain. Life in estuaries must be able to adjust to the varying conditions of the area, including fluctuations in salinity, temperature, and the direction and intensity of the current. You might even think that the amount of life in such places is minimal. However, the contrary holds true—estuaries actually teem with living things that are able to survive in an environment of continuous change. Estuaries happen to be one of the most fertile and liveliest places on earth.

This example presents an opportunity for a shift in our mindset toward change. We human beings should be able to survive—if not thrive—in the constantly changing environment in which we live.

Being cognizant of the fact that change is a natural part of life will help you be prepared for unplanned changes. No, we cannot anticipate some occurrences, but we can have a mindset that will help us adapt to and manage change when it arises.

Multiple Entries onto, Exits from, and Reentries onto Smooth, Paved Roads

Although our life's journey does follow that elusive smooth, paved road from time to time, during periods of life transition we find that we have exited that easy-to-travel path and are now trying to make our way on an unpaved surface. Even more challenging, we might enter a muddy, slippery track and find ourselves struggling hard to get out of it. At such times, we may even come to a complete standstill.

However, there is always the possibility of reentering the smooth, paved road. The manner in which we handle transition periods when we are off that easy surface will determine how fast and via which route we can reenter it.

In essence, our lives consist of periods when we are journeying on smooth, paved roads, periods when we exit onto muddy paths, and then periods when we journey on a new smooth, paved road. We undergo multiple entries, exits, and reentries as we make our journey in life.

On the Issue of Change Readiness

I am always amused when I remember how the world was charged with preparedness for any changes that the millennial year 2000—Y2K—could bring. There was such great anticipation in the air. In particular, preparations were made for possible utility system breakdown. Computer systems were based on the binary system, so the idea that the figures 2000 might be translated into something uninterpretable and cause dysfunction to the utility operations that we so depend on was really scary.

Utilities, other big corporations, and governmental bodies tasked committees with developing preparedness plans. This preparedness issue was extended to all and sundry as news media conveyed information about precautions people should take. One of the measures recommended was that each household should have at least a few weeks' supply of food, water, and other necessary amenities stored up.

Suffice to say that many of the catastrophic predictions did not come to pass—at least not in the general populace. That was a great relief! We all sailed through the arrival of Y2K mostly untouched. However, huge lessons can be learned from the experience. The core one is that we should be prepared to handle changes in general by taking on a change-ready position. When you are in a state of change readiness, you are poised for managing change as opposed to just the outcomes of change. It is a state of being proactive rather than reactive.

Ask yourself:

- Do I resist or ignore change?
- Do I go with the flow of change?

Your answers indicate your current state of change readiness.

Prepare for Unplanned Entries onto the Muddy Tracks of Transitions

Having established that some transitions are within your control and predictable while others are not, the question is: how do you prepare for life transitions in general?

A truck driver traveling on a smooth, paved road always needs to be prepared for an unplanned event. He needs to carry along an extra tire, a compass, a map, a jack, a jump-starter cable, a shovel, a flashlight, rain gear, and an umbrella. Also useful are extra personal items such as clothing and some food and water.

What do you need to carry along with you as you travel on your smooth, paved road so you can be prepared for an unplanned entry onto a muddy track? Here is a useful list of items:

- The right mindset—one that is cognizant of the fact that even though life is settled for now, changes can happen at any time
- A good attitude—if change does happen, it is the way you react to it that determines the outcome
- An active mind for storing up resources you might need if change does happen

- A proactive poise that uses periods of stability to nurture your body, keep in good shape, and feed your spirit; when change comes, you can tap into that reserve of strength, especially at the beginning of the transition

- Willingness to increase your ability to adapt to change by injecting doses of change into your routine

Regarding this last point about purposely changing your day-to-day routine, you might try to:

- Surprise yourself by taking alternative routes to work

- Volunteer your professional services and go on a three-month sabbatical to a country with a different culture from yours

- Switch household responsibilities with your spouse for a period of time

- Add something new to your menu

- Devise new ways of doing things, such as creating a new rule (or modifying an existing one) for saving money, and follow the new approach for some time

- Become friends with someone from a different culture

Your general horizon of day-to-day living will be broadened by these simple acts, and you will be in a better position for embracing changes that come your way.

You Are Not Alone

In upcoming chapters I will describe what happens when life transitions or career changes put you on an unpaved path or, even more challenging, on a slippery, muddy track.

To illuminate the concepts of wisdom to get unstuck and power to move on, we will periodically take a look at the lives of six individuals who are experiencing various kinds of life transitions.

Meet Elena

Elena is a survivor of Hurricane Katrina, which destroyed her native New Orleans. Having lost almost every material possession she could lay claim on—including the local diner that she owned and operated—Elena faces the most traumatic of personal disasters. She is one of the residents moved to Chicago for rehabilitation there, so on top of her long list of transitions Elena also has to experience relocation to a new city.

When Elena's diner went down with the hurricane, more than just the business space and her equipment were lost. Also erased was the very idea of a local diner, where people from the neighborhood came for breakfast before heading to their workplaces. It was a terrible blow. Amidst all the turmoil, Elena did not initially know who had survived or who had not. When she learns later that one of her chefs and one waitress did not make it, she experiences two more huge losses.

Elena suffers a traumatic compendium of losses—personal, career, business, community, social connections, and so on. Her whole world is altogether knocked down. Where is she to start in gathering all the shattered pieces together?

Meet Savannah

Savannah was really happy and excited when she married Fred, the love of her life, just after graduating from college. They had great plans for their future and started a family soon after their marriage. In her career at a pharmaceutical company, Savannah was lucky to have a family-friendly work environment. She enjoyed adequate maternity leaves after the births of both their son and daughter.

In the fifth year of her marriage Savannah was promoted to the position of senior medical representative. She was elated with this new role, which was the career path she had envisaged. With Fred's support she was able to take on the additional travel that her new job required. Fred's career was more flexible and they decided to get some help with household chores and raising the kids.

But in their tenth year of marriage, Savannah and Fred's marriage breaks apart. Fred files for a divorce from what seems out of nowhere. Suddenly, Savannah's smooth, paved road turns into an unpaved, muddy track that she never anticipated.

Meet Harry

Harry has lived a successful life both as a family man and in his career as a college professor. He has lived through a number of challenging diversions from his smooth, paved road, but somehow has always managed to recover and get back on track. Sometimes this restarting of his journey has involved taking different routes from where he was going before the diversions, but in the end he has managed to enjoy more periods of smooth, paved roads in these new directions.

However, just into his retirement years, Harry's spouse of forty years, Debra, passes away. Harry is devastated. None of the previous diversions he has taken into narrow, unpaved roads compare with this. Harry feels like this is the muddiest of all the tracks he has ever entered. The situation is compounded because Harry was trying to adjust to life as a retired person just when this new life-changing event happens. Will Henry ever travel on a smooth, paved road again?

Meet Paul

Paul has been a successful car salesman for almost twenty years. In fact, he started in the trade as a shop assistant in the local car dealership straight out of high school. He never planned to stay in the business this long—his original intention had been to save up for college and then take a professional course that would lead to a job with higher pay. However, that did not happen. Instead, he had stayed in the automotive industry, gotten married, and started raising a family.

Paul met a number of challenges in his career as he progressed, but he kept at it and gradually rose to the position of car salesman in a new dealership that opened a few years into his married life. Paul's wife, Kate, also has a good job as a media representative at the local TV station and is able to supplement the family income. All of a sudden, however, Kate develops severe lower back and hip pain. Her doctor initially recommends conservative treatments, but when these fail Kate has to undergo hip surgery. The whole scenario around the care and treatment of her condition eventually leads to a cutback in her job hours. Paul's job at the car dealership also faces a possible cutback. Paul's smooth, paved road is dramatically turning into an unpaved, muddy path.

Meet Diane

Diane has enjoyed robust health ever since her childhood. Born to athletic parents, she inherited the habits of good exercise—a lifestyle she continued even after leaving home and starting her own business venture.

Although she never married, Diane kept in close contact with her family, who live not too far away from her. Having an outgoing personality, Diane also made a number of close friends and associates while building her business.

Now in her late thirties, Diane is diagnosed with lupus, an ailment that affects many organs of the body. She learns that the disease may affect her skin, joints, kidneys, and brain, and that it often goes on for a long time and presently has no cure.

The disease significantly impairs Diane's ability to perform her job functions. It also impacts other areas of her life.

She can hardly keep up and maintain her composure for a long period of time. Normal day-to-day activities like having dinner out with friends become heavy tasks. The smooth, paved road that Diane had been journeying on has suddenly turned into a sticky, muddy trail.

Meet Ryan

Ryan has overcome many childhood physical issues and, despite all odds, has grown up into a responsible young man. After managing to finish his computing education at a technical college and obtain the necessary industry certifications, Ryan gets his first job with a local start-up firm. Although it is only a part-time position to start, there is the opportunity to move into a full-time position after a probationary period of six months. Ryan is enjoying every minute of his new career. His relationship with a local girl is also getting serious.

When Ryan suffers a terrible injury in a work-related accident, it reopens previous issues he had dealt with during his childhood. Despite all attempts at treatment and surgery, Ryan is confined to a wheelchair. The doctors inform him that chances are slim that he will ever regain full use of his legs. Ryan's smooth, paved road has drastically changed into a muddy path with huge potholes.

Wisdom Tips

Life is defined by change and change gives birth to life.

Unanticipated changes are like transitioning from the smooth highways to the unpaved roads of life.

Power Tips

Periods of emotional crisis are like paved roads full of bumps. Such roads are difficult to travel. However, when managed properly, a positive outcome of personal growth could result.

A right mindset that recognizes that changes can happen at any time is a vital tool in a change-readiness package.

PHASE 2

STUCK!

STUCK!

Phase 2 describes the stage of transition where you are now stuck. It covers your initial attempts to reverse the situation (denial), your desperate efforts to undo whatever was done (anger), and your gradual realization that you are well and truly stuck (acceptance).

In this phase we will discuss the questions:

- Where am I? (Chapter 2)
- How did I get here? (Chapter 3)
- Who am I in this present condition? (Chapter 4)

These three questions are vital for you to answer in your present situation. Without going through this phase, it may be difficult to get unstuck. In fact, your ability to get unstuck and the means and manner for doing so depend on your recognition of where you are now, how you got here, and your sense of identity in the current situation.

This phase is challenging because it may be difficult for you to interact or deal with fellow human beings. You may suspend many day-to-day activities either due to a sheer lack of interest and/or a lack of emotional strength to carry them out. Many things could come to a standstill. You are plagued by many negative emotions that come up due to the sudden change in your circumstances. You may feel lonely, sad, angry, and even depressed that your expectations have not been met.

These challenges are based mainly on the fact that this is the initial phase of your transition. We human beings are creatures of habit, and we try as much as possible to stay in our comfort zones. The stuck phase is the one in which you have been suddenly jolted out of that comfort zone and thrown onto an unpaved muddy, slippery path. At worst you are experiencing a total standstill, something you are not familiar with.

The stuck phase is not a place you want to stay in for any period of time. With respect to comfort and ease, the earlier you can get out of this phase, the better. However, transition periods are the actual periods of growth, and they do take time. It is best to use this period to your advantage.

Take time to dig into the questions I pose throughout the chapters in this section. Your discovery process during this phase will solidify your ability to get unstuck, get liberated, and move forward. Be ready to take the lessons you learn in this phase to move forward on a new paved road when you are ready.

Chapter 2

WHERE AM I?

In the previous chapter I elaborated on what life looks like for you when you are traveling on that elusive smooth, paved road. I then went on to discuss how life's unexpected changes force you to move out from that comfortable, predictable surface onto an untarred path and then onto a muddy, slippery track that is challenging to navigate.

The present chapter deals with your first reaction when your smooth, high-speed journey is diverted into a difficult, slow-speed one that may even come to a standstill in extreme conditions. This is the stage when you recognize that a change has happened to you and you experience your first set of human reactions to it, such as anger, denial, and maybe more anger when you recognize that the change is real and things are no longer the way they used to be.

The Truck That Got Stuck in the Muddy Track

Brian is traveling on a smooth, paved road in his fairly new truck, and is enjoying all aspects of his journey. He had chosen to drive his truck rather than his other vehicle because the truck had more luxury features and, since he was all alone, it seemed the right thing to do. He is driving on cruise control and music from one of his favorite artists is blasting from his sound system. He is just calculating how long it will be before he arrives at his destination when, suddenly, he notices that the well-paved road has disappeared and he is on a narrow, untarred road. Even before he can comprehend it, the untarred road changes further into a muddy track. "What is going on?" Brian wonders. "Where in the world am I?"

In analyzing the questions, Brian looks around his new location. Straight ahead, all he can see is a stretch of muddy path. He checks his rearview and side mirrors and tries to pin down his whereabouts. After a few minutes of checking, he realizes that there is no traffic coming in or out of the area. It is completely isolated. Sheer recognition comes upon him. "Ah! I am alone in the middle of nowhere. The stretch of track ahead is muddy."

Then it starts to dawn on him slowly. He is not in a dream world. His situation is real. His truck is in the middle of a muddy track and there is a problem here. He proceeds to the stage of recognition that sudden change has come upon him. Brian is now aware that things are no longer what they used to be. His journey has been diverted.

Stuck? That can't be true!

Brian's initial recognition triggers an immediate reaction that is not properly thought through. He pumps on the gas in a bid to accelerate and move out quickly before he gets trapped in the situation. It doesn't work. The engine just revs up and the tires spin. He twists the steering wheel this way and that way, trying hard without much thinking to get the truck moving whichever way. But no, the truck will not move.

He tries a few more maneuvers, but they just make things worse. The tires sink even deeper in the mud track. Brian unleashes his anger, shouting at no one in particular. Then more recognition sinks in, and he acknowledges that his truck is not going to move in this muddy path. He is indeed stuck!

Brian then has a fit of denial. Stuck? No, that cannot be true. He gets out and tries to push the truck from the rear all by himself. "That will not work," he finally says to himself.

In fact, all his attempts to get unstuck are just making the truck sink deeper into the mud. Things are not working. He is stuck, stuck, stuck!

Moving from confused to less confused to clarity

After a moment of calming down, Brian is able to think more clearly. He decides to assess the situation under the truck. Bending over, he checks the position of the wheels relative to the muddy track and to the ruts he had created when revving the engine. He looks to see how deep the muddy tracks are and if there are any potholes around the area where his truck now rests.

With this understanding of the position of the wheels and his truck as a whole, Brian is a little reassured that there might be a way out. As he comes more to himself, he realizes this is what he should have done in the first place.

He now decides to check his bearings relative to the original smooth, paved road he had been traveling before his truck was suddenly diverted. He takes out his compass to determine the direction of the muddy track. He unfolds his map to see whether he can pinpoint his location. "This information will be needed," he thinks, "if I need to call for assistance."

Get the Confusion Out

Brian's first set of reactions to his truck's entry into a muddy track depicts what happens to you at the onset of a life or career-changing event. When you are suddenly plunged into the muddy path of a transition, you tend to enter a confused state. You may even be in a state of shock. Since the change is a new event, you may not be very cognizant of what has happened.

As human beings we are conditioned to having a fight-or-flight reaction to any dangerous or unwanted event. So it is natural to put up a struggle when you face a sudden change. Adrenaline is released into your system and, without thinking about it, you just kick at the change to get rid of it as quickly as possible. However, after a few attempts, you begin to acknowledge that something is indeed different in your situation. No mere kicking or fighting will alter the condition.

At this stage, confusion sets in. You are puzzled as to why what used to be is no longer so. You become perplexed that what used to work is no longer working. Depending on the complexity of the situation, you may become bewildered. You may also feel embarrassed, disoriented, or awkward.

No matter how your confusion about the change is expressed, you need to become clear about what has happened and where you are in your life's journey as a result of the change. You need to assess your situation and recognize the things you have lost. You need to identify factors that are no longer the same. And you need to know what things are new in your present situation.

However, it is not always easy, especially at the onset of a transition, to have the clear mind required to recognize or assess what has changed. To get enough mental space to see things clearly, there needs to be a form of mourning, an expression of your grief. This is a stage of going back and forth, from recognition to anger to denial and back again.

Express Your Feelings about the Change You Perceive

While you are in the mourning stage, it is important that you express your feelings about the situation. One way to express your dissatisfaction about the sudden change or calamity is to verbalize your emotions. Talk about the changes you perceive to people within your easy reach when you first recognize something has happened. Depending on the change you have experienced, this first set of people may or may not be people you already know. Regardless, it is still important to express your initial feelings.

Continue to talk about the change you have come to recognize to discerning people who have your interests at heart, such as family members and close friends. On its own, voicing your feelings can relieve some of the stress you are experiencing. In addition, when you express your feelings to a discerning ear it may help that individual understand what you are experiencing and offer you ways out of the situation.

When you are voicing your feelings about a sudden upheaval in your life, it may help to ask yourself:

- Am I angry?
- Am I confused? Do I need more information to clarify my situation?
- Am I afraid?
- Do I feel like I am losing the ability to manage the situation?
- Do I feel overwhelmed?
- Does it feel like I am carrying a heavy weight on my shoulders?
- Do I feel like I am walking in place, going through the motions but not getting anywhere?
- Do I feel trapped or pinned down?
- Does it feel like I am in the middle of nowhere?

Venting is a good tool for releasing bottled-up emotions that may be keeping you from understanding your current position.

Understand Where You Are and Determine Your Bearings

Using any of the above means and/or combinations of them to express your feelings about your transition will ease your stress and help you come to an understanding of where you are in your life's journey.

Brian, the driver of the truck that got stuck in the muddy path, was able to get an understanding of where he was in his journey through two means. First, he assessed the position of the truck and the alignment of the wheels relative to the depth of the muddy tracks. This was a localized (micro) description of his exact position. Second, Brian assessed his bearings—his position relative to the rest of the world (a macro description).

During this initial phase of your transition it is helpful that you determine your present position at both the micro and macro levels. Your micro position may be in a deep pothole on a muddy path. Maybe no one was with you when you entered the pothole. Perhaps a few people eventually pass by and one or two of these even splash water on you unintentionally, creating more challenges on top of the existing ones. Having a sense of your exact position will help you start to figure out a way out.

Your macro position will help you identify how the direction of your journey has been impacted by the change you experienced. Maybe you were going north before and now your new direction is northeast. This knowledge is important as you will need it to map out a new route (as will be discussed in later chapters). Just as Brian the truck driver tried to figure out his bearings by using a compass, you may need to deliberate on where you are with reference to the community around you so you can figure out a way back into it.

Your macro position will also determine the time you will need to get to where you were going before you got diverted or to get to a new destination—and, therefore, the type of plan you now need to achieve your goals.

Savannah Has to Get the Confusion out about Her Divorce

Savannah, introduced in Chapter 1, is the mother of two who receives a divorce filing from her husband of ten years. When Savannah first gets news about the divorce, she is shocked and altogether confused. In fact, she shakes all over for a couple of days. "This can't be happening to me," she says. Then she goes into a rage and shouts at everyone who tries to talk to her. Finally, she realizes the best option is to take time off work to think things through.

She tries to identify exactly what has happened to her, but she can't seem to come to terms with it. She goes through a denial stage where she convinces herself that Fred, her husband, is still there for her. "Maybe this is only a nightmare or some weird dream," she tells herself. "This can't be true."

For Savannah, being clear on her present position or status means being clear in her mind that she is no longer married to Fred. Understanding that she is no longer a married woman is essential to understanding the many implications of this fact. For instance, she will no longer be living in the same house with Fred. She can no longer refer to him as her husband in any social circle or legal documents. She can no longer have all of those long-term dreams and plans that they previously had for their marriage. She and Fred now have to come to some agreement on custody of their two children. Her finances can no longer be mixed with Fred's. And so the list goes on.

Paul Has to Understand His New Position

Paul, the car salesman introduced in Chapter 1, eventually loses his job when the dealership he was working for goes through a downsizing. Paul is devastated. The thing he greatly feared has now come upon him, and it is all too much. First it was the problem with his wife Kate's back and hip, which led to her having surgery and a cutback in the number of hours she could work. Now his job is gone, too. Why now? Why him?

Paul is confused. He experiences the range of possible emotions in reaction to his job loss. He feels overwhelmed and trapped. But to get unstuck, he needs to know exactly what is going on in his life's journey.

A number of days after losing his job, Paul realizes he has to understand his present position and come up with a new plan. The first understanding that comes to him is that he will no longer be going to the dealership to log in for work. Relative to the rest of the world of employed people, his position has changed. When it comes to his micro position— his family—his ability to bring home income to support their finances has also changed.

Be Clear on Your Present Position

Brian was able to define his location not only with reference to the rest of the world, but also with reference to his micro locality—the finer details of the change he has experienced. The alignment of his wheels in the muddy track is one of those fine details. Knowing the alignment will help him decide which way to twist the wheels to get his truck moving in the direction he desires. It will help him determine the initial steps he needs to take to get out of the immediate rut. Once he gets out of that immediate locality, he will then be able to address more global factors such as where he is now relative to the rest of the world.

For life and career transitions, the fine details will refer to how the transition has altered your family setting, your inner circle of influence, and your day-to-day activities. These fine details are important because they are factors in your immediate environment that you deal with on a daily basis. Changes in these factors significantly impact your stress level and ability to adapt to more global changes.

Give Yourself Permission to Mourn Your Loss

When you do come to recognize that things are no longer as they used to be, it is necessary to start grieving the things you have identified as lost. The form of your grieving is up to you, but it is a helpful step toward acquiring sanity and strength for your transition days.

Savannah needs to take time to mourn the loss of her marriage and all the factors associated with it. She needs to mourn the loss of the previously established stability of her family. In this initial period, mourning may be mixed with anger and denial as Savannah goes back and forth, trying to restore what was lost.

Paul needs to give himself permission to mourn the years of work he put in at the car dealership. He needs to grieve the loss of the camaraderie he had enjoyed at his former workplace and the circle of friends he had formed through his associations. Even the journey to work every morning, which featured scenery he enjoys, is no longer part of his life (at least in the initial stage of the transition). He needs to grieve that too.

Sanity and Strength Are Important at the Onset of a Transition

Sanity and strength have important roles to play at this stage of your transition. In a confused state, your mind is not very stable. You go through cycles of recognition, anger, and denial. You need sanity and strength to take in what has happened, process it in your brain, and digest it. In ruminating back and forth over what has happened, you may come to initial recognition and some understanding of the change. More reflection and deliberation may help you identify what exactly you have lost. Thinking over the event will help you nail down which factors in your life are no longer the same as they used to be.

The process to achieve clarity on where you are and which factors have changed in your life may take some time. Expressing your grief in concrete ways, such as talking to family members and friends, will help you become clear on your new position. Outlining factors that you have lost as a result of the life-changing event will help you move from a perplexed state to one of greater clarity and understanding. This understanding (or at least an initial perception of it) will help you analyze how you got into the present situation. This issue of discovering how you arrived on the muddy path is the topic of the next chapter.

Wisdom Tips

Feeling embarrassed, disoriented, or awkward is a natural part of the set of reactions at the onset of when you first experience a diversion from your smooth paved road to one that is unpaved.

Getting the confusion out is highly important so as to become aware of the new 'new' in your circumstances.

Give yourself permission to mourn your loss. Expressing your grief in concrete ways, such as talking to family members and friends, will help you become clear on your new position.

Power Tips

Venting is a good tool for releasing bottled-up emotions that may be keeping you from understanding your current position impacted by the transition.

Understanding where you are in terms of your immediate environment and your bearings in relation to a more global picture will help you in obtaining more clarity as to how the transition has impacted you.

Chapter 3

HOW DID I GET HERE?

The previous chapter highlighted the importance of understanding your new position as defined by the life-changing events you have experienced. Having been able to define where you are in your current situation, your mind, which is still struggling to accept the change, questions, "How did I get here? How could this have happened?"

How Could This Have Happened?

Brian, the driver of the nice truck that suddenly entered a muddy track, ponders his situation. "I was having a nice smooth journey. How in the world did I get here? How could this have happened?"

Brian takes some time to analyze these questions. First, he recognizes that landing on this muddy track was not his fault. No, he had heeded all the road signs, had kept his truck in good shape for driving, and had well-maintained tires. He had filled the truck with fuel before starting his journey. He had even listened to the weather forecast, and everything seemed to be clear in the direction of his journey. He had been totally prepared for his originally planned journey. What he had been unprepared for was this sudden diversion into a muddy track.

After going through cycles of anger and denial, you may gradually come to terms with the fact that the change you have experienced is real. It takes courage to move from a stage of asking, "Why me? Why now?" to a stage where you can begin to look critically at your situation and ask, "How did I get here?"

When you are able to ask this last question, it signifies that you are making some shifts in your transition journey. As there are no fixed lines across the stages, when you are at this stage you might still go back and forth between denial and acceptance. However, taking the initial step to assess how you got into the situation is a step forward in the right direction.

What Caused the Entry onto the Muddy Track?

Changes are varied in terms of whether they are natural, induced, forced upon you, or created by you. The way to analyze how you got into the situation varies accordingly.

For our truck driver, Brian, his sudden entry into the muddy track was not something he had created. It happened abruptly and unexpectedly. If Brian had ignored a grim weather forecast, he would have to acknowledge the role he had played in landing on the muddy track. If Brian had been distracted in his driving by the use of handheld devices, or if he had ignored other rules of safe driving such as exceeding a safe speed, he would have to admit his personal responsibility for causing the transition. If he had known that his chosen road had many contours that had not been well traveled or well mapped, then he would have to take responsibility for the decision he had made to take that route.

However many life-changing events are not laden with these kinds of parameters. Many events that land us on muddy pathways are changes forced upon us. Taking stock of how you got into the situation does not mean you are always to take full blame for what has happened. To the contrary, it means you will be able to objectively check if your personal factors contributed to the event and, if so, what those factors are. This stock taking will help you define the steps (at least the initial ones) you might need to take to get out of your current situation.

Questioning "How did I get here?" and "How could this have happened?" is an indication that you are looking for answers. You are searching for some form of meaning to relate to what has happened. This quest for meaning and purpose is at the heart of the quest for sanity and strength to get unstuck and move forward from the change.

Ryan Needs to Define the Cause of His Life-changing Event

In Chapter 1 you met Ryan, who was laden with multiple issues of transition within a short period of time. When Ryan is told by doctors that he will likely never use his legs again, it is the most devastating news he has ever heard. After overcoming his initial shock, Ryan is in a confused state for several days. When he is able to clarify that the situation about his legs is real, Ryan goes back and forth in cycles of anger and denial. He is on an intense quest for sanity and strength to overcome the challenges of his present situation.

Considering the many obstacles he has already had to face in his life, all Ryan can ask at the beginning of this new transition is, "Why me again? Aren't those past experiences enough? Why do I have to face another physical challenge?" It takes time for Ryan to digest what has happened. Gradually, Ryan is able to express his feelings verbally. He talks about the fact that he is confined to a wheelchair. When he is able to muster enough courage, Ryan asks himself, "How did this happen? How did I get here?" He is able to look objectively at the incident in his mind's eye. He remembers what happened to him at work on the day of the accident. He recalls how he was crossing over from one building to another wing at his workplace for an appointment. He was crossing the lane when a delivery truck driver had backed out and, not knowing Ryan was there, had hit him. The more Ryan thinks about it, the more he remembers.

With this recollection, Ryan starts to talk to people around him about the events on that day. He narrates it many times to as many people who will listen. The more he talks about it, the more clarity comes to his mind. Then he takes to the Internet and starts blogging about his experience. He gets responses from readers of his blog through this outlet. Ryan finds that voicing his grief and writing about it is, in fact, helping him deal with the situation.

Define the Stimulus of the Transition

Depending on the loss you have experienced, trying to describe what caused the transition may or may not be easy. For natural disasters that are totally out of your control, it is quite straightforward to nail down the stimulus. For people like Elena who lived in a city invaded by a hurricane, suffice it to say that the hurricane was the stimulus of the loss they experienced.

For someone who loses a job, the stimulus can be mixed. If an individual works with a company that downsizes due to a recession and he is given a six-month termination package, the stimulus for that transition is the company's internal reorganization (and the economy). However, for someone who loses her job due to career malpractice or lack of productivity on the job, the stimulus for that transition cannot be put on the workplace. That person will have to describe why she lacked productivity and the factors that led to that issue.

Facing facts about such stimuli will help you not only address the loss but also draw out an action plan for reentering a new smooth, paved road. The plan might include steps to address issues such as work ethics, behavioral patterns, and possible upgrading of skills.

The change you are experiencing might have been caused by a series of events. These events could have happened suddenly within a short period of time, or they might have been a long time in the making. Whichever is the case, describing the events, especially the crucial ones, will help you clear away even more confusion and achieve new understanding about your current situation. This will help you come to terms with your new circumstances.

Harry Narrates the Story of His Loss Many Times Over

Harry is the recently retired college professor introduced in Chapter 1 who lost his wife of forty years. Harry was trying hard to adjust to his life as a retired man just before his wife's death occurred. Being a hardworking person who put a lot of himself into his career as a college professor, Harry had found it hard to just sit at home and do nothing. At the time of his retirement, Debra, his wife, was still working full time and was not due for retirement for another five years, so Harry had checked out options for some part-time engagement to keep him fulfilled. A former colleague who had retired earlier had pointed him in the direction of an e-learning project that Harry could easily engage in from home.

It was while on a trip to visit the head office of the company spearheading the e-learning project that Harry received an urgent phone call. Debra had been rushed to the hospital due to a strange infection. Try hard as the medical team did to make her better, Debra's illness got worse. She passed away a few days after her admission.

Harry is shattered. Going through cycles of shock, anger, and denial, Harry keeps asking, "Why? Why now? Why Debra?" He feels devastated that he had not been able to help her. He bargains with himself, promising that he will do anything that is required if only Debra could get another chance. In his grieving process, Harry narrates to people all the events leading up to the death of his wife. He shows people pictures of Debra. He talks about how she had been in good health up until that terrible infection. He talks about those last few days and how her death had been so sudden. Harry expresses his grief in this verbal way and through other means.

Express Your Feelings about What Caused the Transition

Just as it was for Harry, it is important for you to express your grief. You might have started expressing it when you first recognized that things were no longer the same as they used to be. Now that you have identified what caused the transition, it is pertinent to continue to express your grief by talking about the stimulus of your transition in more tangible ways.

Tell as many people as will listen about how the change happened, the process that led to it, and the events surrounding it. Whether you have experienced the loss of physical objects, a close relationship, or aspects of your health or physical fitness, the process of relating the story to others is a good outlet for your grief.

Ask yourself questions that will help nail down your attitude about the transition and its cause(s).

- What do I regret doing that might have caused the transition, or what do I regret not doing that might have prevented it?

- What do I resent about my current situation?

- What do I feel bitter about or have hard feelings about?

Your regrets could include things that you wish you could have done before the change happened. They may have nothing to do with the change, but could be impossible to do now that the change has happened. For instance, if you had wanted to go on a special trip with your spouse and the life-changing event was the loss of that spouse, you have also lost the opportunity for that trip (at least with your spouse). Even if you still go where you had planned, the trip may not be as meaningful.

You may also regret the way you did something before the change happened. Looking back, you may wish you had done something differently.

Issues that you may resent could relate to the stimulus or the manner in which the change happened. Expressing your feelings about things you resent is important. It will help you avoid getting stuck in the guilt lane on that issue in the future. It will also release you from inadvertently taking blame for something that may have been totally out of your control.

Below are some other methods for expressing your feelings about the change you are experiencing.

Keep a journal about your experience

Writing your thoughts down in a journal or elsewhere will help you release stored-up feelings of anger about the change you have recognized and the stimulus that induced it. You might use a hard-copy journal and block out a regular time for recording your feelings each day. Or, if you are comfortable with the idea, you might journal online in the form of a blog or other social media in which you can express your feelings to an online community of friends. Whichever method you decide to employ, journaling will help you get out the confusion about your situation. The process of putting your thoughts into writing serves to release some of the negative emotions you may be experiencing. It will help you clear the mental space you may need to see clearly into your circumstance.

Join a support group

Another helpful way to verbalize your feelings about your life-changing event is through the use of a support group or forum of other individuals who are in transitions similar to the one you are experiencing. Opportunities for telling your story abound in such groups. The ability to talk freely without any blaming fingers or restrictions will serve as a good support for you. In addition, listening to other people express their own grief reassures you that you are not alone in your situation.

Use community support services

Community support services are very helpful in cases where you do not have friends or family close by when you experience a sudden turn in your life's journey. Public information centers and libraries have lists of support resources in your community. You may decide, for example, to sign up for a one-on-one session with a mentor and/or community leader who can offer a listening ear and help you through the process of grieving your loss.

A Rude Interruption or an Avenue for Growth?

The sections above dealt with identifying what caused the transition you are experiencing as well as how you can express your grief about your loss. These are important processes for you to move forward during a life transition. Another important parameter to pay attention to during this period is your mindset toward the transition as a whole. Your attitude will direct the outcome of your transition as you move from grieving to taking action for entering a new smooth, paved road.

Since your life's journey was going smoothly on the paved road, the diversion onto a sticky, muddy path can seem like a nuisance. Imagine if your favorite show was playing on the big screen and someone interrupted it by turning off the electric power. "This is absurd!" you might yell. "How can you do that?" When you realize the power is not coming back on anytime soon, you may go on to say something like, "At least you should have warned me." Yes, the shutting off of the electric power at that moment was not only an interruption but was rude and impolite because you were not forewarned.

No one likes rude interruptions, especially when they are in the middle of an activity they were enjoying and having great success with. Thus, when you consider the life-changing event you are going through, it is natural to regard it as a rude interruption to your normal life. However, maintaining that kind of perspective could continue to fuel your negative emotions of anger and bitterness. It is more realistic to take on a perspective that is diametrically opposite to this view.

Instead of counting the change as an impolite disturbance, consider it as an opportunity to grow as a person. With the right attitude, you can develop maturity while managing this transition. Yes, it is true that you are angry and greatly dissatisfied about your current situation. However, learn that you can channel this anger into a positive route. When you do this, you are redirecting your energy toward achieving goals that will help you change the issue you are dissatisfied with into something that brings you great satisfaction.

Change is indeed a paradox. It offers great opportunities for learning more about yourself and at the same time frustrates your attempts to create a stable and predictable world.

Consider the transition as a challenge, one that you can muster all that it takes to overcome. Recognize that walking through this period may stretch you as a person, but the victory on the other end of the journey is worth all the effort you can put into the actual walk. This kind of mindset and perspective will help you acquire the sanity and strength to manage your transition successfully. When managed well, the transition will be like a stepping stone toward a new paved road.

In addition, look at your transition as a period where you can develop an attitude of resilience that will enable you to stay on top of your challenges. This attitude will be of great use not just for this one transition but for other challenges you may meet in the whole of your life's journey.

Understand Your Attitude toward the Stimulus of the Transition

In addition to your attitude to the transition you are experiencing, your attitude toward the stimulus that caused it is also important. Take time to ask yourself the following questions, which will help you see how you view the stimulus in the big picture of your life-changing event:

- Am I attaching too much blame to it?

The stimulus or factor that caused the transition is only that: a stimulus.

- Am I using the stimulus to wallow in self-pity?

- Am I using the stimulus to be re-victimized about my experience—the event itself?

You do not need to hang on to the stimulus or signs and images of it. You need to recognize the stimulus for what it is: only a stimulus.

Ryan, the young man who lost the use of his legs, identified that his work accident was the stimulus for the present transition he was facing. Simply put, if he had not had that accident, he would not have had leg surgery, nor would he be confined to a wheelchair today. If Ryan is to move forward with his life's journey, he needs to face facts about the stimulus of the transition. Ryan should not keep clothing that event and feeding it in his mind. Yes, he needs to talk about it and grieve the loss of the use of his legs. However, he does not need to stay stuck with the stimulus—the events of that day.

It is important to have a mindset that does not overrate the stimulus of your transition. Rather, it is helpful to acknowledge what the stimulus is, recognize how it has induced the change, and understand it for what it really is: only a stimulus. The transition itself is what you will need to work on. The process of acquiring the wisdom to get unstuck and the power to move on is of utmost importance. You need to downgrade the stimulus in your mind's eye and upgrade your attempts at getting the sanity and strength you need to manage your transition well.

Continue to Give Yourself Permission to Mourn

As mentioned in Chapter 2, the recognition stage is a good place to start allowing yourself to mourn what you have lost due to the changes. When you have moved through recognition and gradual acceptance and have been able to take stock as described in this chapter, do not neglect the aspect of mourning. Continue to allow yourself to mourn in ways that seem best to you. Do not try and hide under a shadow of false composure. It is better to be broken and then heal over the course of time than to have a cover-up that all is well when all is not actually well.

Identifying what caused you to enter the muddy path is an important step toward acceptance of the change. This, in turn, is required for overcoming any inertia the change might be causing and thereby finding means of getting unstuck. However, as discussed above, at this stage of the transition you may still be going back and forth between denial and acceptance. This is because the change has had an impact not only on your environment, but also on you as a person— your real self.

Therefore, it is equally important to identify the implication of the transition on your sense of self at this moment. It is vital to understand how the change has affected who you really are in your current situation. The next chapter addresses this issue.

Wisdom Tips

Your attitude will direct the outcome of your transition as you move from grieving to taking action for entering a new smooth, paved road.

With the right attitude, you can develop maturity while managing your transition.

Putting your thoughts into writing serves to release some of the negative emotions you may be experiencing. It will help you clear the mental space you may need to see clearly into your circumstance.

Power Tips

Express your feelings about things you resent about what caused the transition will help you avoid getting stuck in the guilt lane on that issue in the future.

It will also release you from inadvertently taking blame for something that may have been totally out of your control.

Learn to channel your anger and dissatisfaction about the transition into a positive route. When you do this, you are redirecting your energy toward achieving goals that will help you change the issue you are dissatisfied with into something that brings you great satisfaction.

Chapter 4

WHO AM I IN THIS PRESENT CONDITION?

In the previous chapter I addressed the issue of coming to terms with the fact that you are in a transition. I explained the role of objective analysis and mindset shifts in this process, and highlighted steps such as delineating the cause of the transition and taking on new perspectives. The current chapter describes the effect that life and career transitions can have on your sense of self and your overall identity.

A Stuck Truck or a Stuck Driver?

Brian, the driver of the truck who suddenly found he had been diverted from a nice, smooth, paved road, continues to reflect on his condition. He has assessed his situation and, although he can't figure out how he got into that track, he is now sure that the situation is real. Having accepted that he is actually stuck in the muddy track, a thought quickly flashes in his mind: among the important documents in his wallet is his car insurance company's roadside assistance hotline number.

As quickly as the thought enters his mind, his next reaction is that of withdrawal. He thinks about the process of calling that number; he will have to tell them why he is calling. "What am I supposed to tell them?" he asks himself. "How does it sound to say, 'Hello, my truck got stuck,' or 'I am the driver of a stuck truck'?"

Then it hits him hard. He has suddenly become the driver of a stuck truck. Or is he just a stuck driver? No matter how he twists the words around, the fact is he has a new title to his name. This new label is one he will bear at least until his circumstances change.

Brian does not stop there in his ponderings. He also reflects on how this new designation will affect his life in the future. Will being a stuck driver label him as incompetent? Will he have to admit to everyone that he was a stuck driver? "Uh, this situation has some implications for my future," he admits to himself.

The Effect Life Transitions Have on Your Identity

Life transitions and enormous changes in your circumstances can leave you confused and frustrated. Many of the challenges have their roots in the fact that your identity changes when you are going through a period of transition.

Identity is the set of characteristics that distinguishes an individual from any other individual. It is based on parameters such as skills, relationships, and behavior. During normal times, these parameters tend to remain stable. However, during a transitional period the continuity of one's identity is disrupted.

It does not matter whether the transition is due to a forced change or a natural change or even a change you created—it will still have significant impact on your identity. Changes such as retirement, marriage, parenthood, or grandparenthood are mostly anticipated, but they all still impact who you are. When you intentionally change your career or move across the city or country, you may have some time to think things through before the actual event. You have time to extinguish many doubts you have about such a change because it is in part created by you. Even so, this type of change impacts who you are and who you become. Unexpected or unanticipated changes such as natural disasters, divorce, loss of a loved one, or job loss have an even greater impact.

As you experience these transitions, the loss of continuity in some aspects of your life causes a conflict inside of you. This conflict is based on the difference between who you perceive yourself to be and who your changed circumstance is trying to make you into. This conflict tends to leave you overwhelmed and stuck.

Therefore, it is of utmost importance for you to recognize that you are no longer who you used to be and that you seek to resolve this crisis in your identity. It is important to eliminate the confusion about your social role—an issue at the heart of the crisis in identity. The process of doing this will prepare you for the stage of moving forward.

Identify Factors of Your Old Identity That Were Lost

The change you experience as a result of a life or career transition can be observed in many aspects of your identity:

- Physical self/self-esteem
- Family
- Social
- Community
- Career/intellectual
- Economic
- Spiritual

The degree of impact on each of these areas depends on the type of transition you are going through. Relationship-based transitions such as divorce and loss of a loved one tend to impact many more areas of your life than other types of transitions. This may be the reason why higher stress levels are associated with those types of transitions, as rated by scales such as the Holmes and Rahe scale.

Thomas Holmes and Richard Rahe's Social Re-adjustment Rating Scale[1] attempts to quantify the impact of different stressful events in terms of the extent to which a person would need to readjust their established lifestyle in order to adapt to the situation. On a scale of 1 to 100, the death of a spouse rates as 100, that of a close family relative (other than a spouse) as 63, and that of a close friend as 37. Other relationship-based transitions also rank high on this scale. Divorce, a very traumatic event, rates at 73 while marital separation rates at 65.

Since you are a whole person, segments of your identity cannot be isolated. Therefore, what impacts your family identity will impact other areas of your identity, such as your self-esteem and your identity as a whole.

Here are some examples of how certain life transitions are reflected in the loss in continuity of your identity.

Physical self/self-esteem

If your loss is of a loved one, you are no longer able to interact with the physical presence of that individual. The same holds true in a breakdown of a relationship, such as in divorce or the end of a business partnership. Your self-perceptions are greatly affected by your loss. The loving relationship that used to boost your feelings of worthiness and acceptance is no longer there. This situation impacts your self-esteem.

Your self-esteem is also greatly affected if you lose a job, because who you are is often depicted by what you do to earn a living. When the ability to earn an income or play a significant role in your community is lost, so are your feelings of being capable or worthy.

[1]Thomas Holmes and Richard Rahe. "Social Re-adjustment Rating Scale," *Journal of Psychosomatic Research 11, no. 2 (1967): 213–18.*

Family identity

The death of a member of your family changes the family structure significantly. For instance, when parents undergo a divorce or when a spouse dies, a double-parent family changes to a single-parent one. Family roles filled by the other partner are left unfulfilled.

Social identity

Your social identity is intricately linked to your family and career life. Therefore, changes in the structure of your family and/or career life impact your social status.

When you experience a life-changing event, friends and acquaintances in the places you normally visit may view you differently. This could be reflected in your interactions with a wide range of people such as your dentist, your hairdresser, your accountant, and people at the parties you attend.

Community identity

Your interactions with your neighbors are affected if you lose someone in your family. Members of the community circle to which you and your deceased family member belonged may view you differently.

Career/intellectual identity

After experiencing a job loss, your status of being a career person changes and so does your identity. This career identity is often linked to self-esteem and, thus, a general sense of self.

Retirement also brings about a significant change in your intellectual identity. This is due to the loss of a lifestyle pattern in which you were a "functional" person who contributed to society.

Career changers also experience a significant impact on their identity that is often determined by factors linked to the difference between the old and the new situation. Such factors include societal associations of status, income earning potential, required skill sets, and flexibility patterns.

Economic identity

Transitions such as job loss, death of a partner, divorce, and retirement can have a significant effect on your economic identity and necessitate adjustments in your lifestyle.

Spiritual identity

Marriage has a spiritual component to it. Our work, a means of our creativity, also has a spiritual element. Thus, part of your spiritual self is interwoven with your relationship with your partner or with your work. A transition may alter your spiritual identity and change your desire for spiritual connection.

Temporary or Long-term Impacts on Identity

Brian the truck driver has to accept a new reality. Not only has his situation changed; his identity has changed as well. In Brian's case it may be easy not to worry about this new identity, since it is temporary. Once he gets his truck back on the road it may be easy to erase the fact that he was once a stuck driver for a certain period of time. However, in other life transitions, the identity of the individual is impacted in more profound ways. For instance, it will be a much longer haul for Elena, a survivor of Hurricane Katrina, to resume her life's journey with a new identity.

Elena Feels Like Her Whole Past Has Been Erased

Elena can't even express how she feels in a cogent way. All the physical objects that constituted her past were destroyed by the hurricane. None of the memories she had built in New Orleans could be traced through physical means. She still has those memories stored up in her brain, but the tangible objects of her life are all gone—her family home, her diner where she had served many people breakfast, her church, her sports center, her community center. They are all items of the past. It's earth-shattering!

With this devastating kind of phenomenon, not only has Elena lost her identity in all areas of her life, she has also lost the thread of connection to her past that physical things provide. It feels as if her data set has been deleted from some computer storage bank. Elena needs emotional power to bail herself out of her crisis.

In other people's life-changing events, the individual who loses something can usually go back to a familiar place from the past and use it as a place of mourning and a starting point for healing. This is not the case for Elena and the other survivors of the hurricane. The physical objects are gone forever. As a result, Elena needs an enormously long period of time to grieve her lost identities, seek a new identity with which she can connect with the future, and subsequently move forward with that new identity.

Recognize That Your Lost Identity No Longer Exists

Coming to terms with the fact that the identity you lost is no longer available for your use is an important step in getting unstuck during life transitions (see Chapter 5). You need to recognize that the "you" who was previously traveling on the smooth, paved road no longer exists.

The career person who was the investigative officer at ABC Corporation can no longer bear that title after he loses his job. Not only is the title gone, but the individual can no longer represent the company, carry out business on their behalf, or earn his income through any of those activities. That old person no longer exists. The individual who loses his leg in an accident and is confined to a wheelchair needs to come to terms with the fact that his old self who used to be able to walk or run has stopped existing. That aspect of his identity is gone. And the married woman who gets divorced needs to recognize that she no longer bears the label of Mrs. "B." No, that is the past. She can no longer claim to be Mr. B's wife, and in many cases may no longer legally sign documents on his behalf regarding any entities they previously jointly held.

So, depending on the particular type of transition, some aspects of your former identity, status, and self-image may no longer apply after you have experienced the change.

Mourn Your Lost Identity

Since you can no longer use a lost identity once a change occurs, the best thing you can do is let it go. Let it go? Yes, stop hanging on to it. Release it as a thing of the past. An effective way to say goodbye to a lost identity is to take the time to mourn it.

When you have lost something that is as valuable as an identity, it is helpful to take some time to relive the great memories you created with that identity before it was inadvertently taken from you. Recount the joys and victories you had when that identity still belonged to you. If you are a visually expressive person, try creating a collage of memories of that identity from pictures or images from the past.

To stimulate memories you might want to honor about your lost identity, ask yourself:

- What do I miss most about being the person who had the designation that is now lost?

- What do I miss most about my lost identity?

- If I could keep one thing about my lost identity, what would it be?

After reliving the memories that come up, recognize and acknowledge that your lost identity served you well when you had it. But now that it is no longer there, you will just have to let it go. Take time to say goodbye to it in your mind's eye or, if occasion calls for it, loudly and in a solid, tangible way.

Once you have honored your memories and said your goodbyes, you will be able to shift your position and prepare your mind for the next stage. That next stage will become real as you try to envision living your life without the identity you lost and have just said goodbye to.

Elena, the survivor of Hurricane Katrina, has a long list of things she misses about New Orleans and her life and work there. She talks about how everything was glorious about her former home, but when asked to talk specifically about what she misses about who she was in New Orleans, Elena is able to narrow her list. Interestingly enough, the aspect of her identity that she misses most is how she fed the neighborhood in the morning before they went to work. She misses the neighbors who gathered around her in her local breakfast diner. She misses the role she played in their lives. Unbeknownst to her, she had relished being like a mother to them all as she provided breakfast for them.

Envision a Future without Your Lost Identity

Once you have honored and said goodbye to your old identity, it is necessary to figure out what life will look like without it. Ask yourself:

- What will life look like without my old status?
- What will it be like to live day-to-day without that designation?

This thought-provoking process requires you to be courageous about probing into the future and envisaging what life will be like without something you have lived with, in many cases, for a number of years. However, these are questions that will help you recognize and acknowledge that there is a gap between the old you and the new you who will be living in the future you have envisioned. To bridge that gap you need to seek a new identity for your entry onto a new smooth, paved road. You cannot afford not to have such a new identity.

Diane Finds it Hard to See Her Future Self without Her Lost Identity

Diane, the businesswoman introduced in Chapter 1 who was diagnosed with lupus, considers her new situation. What she misses most about her old identity was her ability to carry out a great number of tasks during the day without getting tired. She had been someone who seemed to run on autopilot as she took on one new task after another. Her friends and close associates had always remarked on this ability and sometimes wished they could function like she did. That kind of report about her no longer holds true with the presence of the disease.

It is very difficult for Diane to see herself as someone who is limited to significantly fewer working hours. Her business venture had been a great part of her identity and she is struggling to envision a future without it. Diane begins a deep search for sanity and strength to overcome the challenges of her present complex situation.

What Will Having This New Designation or Label Mean for Me in the Future?

In the section above I explained the concept of envisaging life without your old identity. An equally important view of the concept lies in the fact that when you lose an old identity, you inadvertently gain a new one. If you lose a job you become a jobless person or a jobseeker. If you lose your spouse through death, you become a widow or widower. If you experience a divorce, you are labeled a divorcé(e).

These societal labels conjure images of helplessness or lost hope. But while you may receive one of these labels when you lose your identity in a life transition, you need to see it as that: a label. It is not equivalent to your whole make-up, which is your *real* identity. Giving too much attachment to that label or designation will not help you move forward. You need to recognize that your attitude to such a label will either make you or continue to break you. You need to transcend the image of that label.

As mentioned above, take time to mourn the lost identity that has resulted in this new label. Then ask yourself the question:

- How will the perception of who I am
  affect my life in the future?

Verbally express your feelings about the perception of who you are due to the change that has happened to you.

You Need a New Identity to Carry You into the Future

You need to accept that you require a new identity to move into the future. Then prepare your mind to search for a new identity that will work for you in your move forward. Although a new identity won't erase the label you receive when you undergo a life transition, it will, when properly developed, provide new designations and status on a new smooth, paved road.

In the last three chapters I discussed key questions that will help you when you have just entered a life or career transition— i.e., when you are in the "stuck" phase. Having recognized where you are due to the change and having identified the factors in your life that have been altered as a result, you went on to analyze what caused the change. Recognizing the stimulus is a necessary process that helps you mourn what you have lost and analyze how the change has affected you as a person. When you come to terms with the changes in your identity due to the transition you are experiencing, you will see the need for a new identity that can help you enter a new smooth, paved road in your life's journey.

All the above processes stimulate discovery when you are in the stuck position. This discovery is essential if you are to move from stuck to unstuck. But what do you really need to do to get unstuck? Which tools do you need to have in place? Answers to these and similar questions are the focus of the next section.

Wisdom Tips

Transitions cause a disruption in the continuity of your identity. The conflict that results tends to leave you overwhelmed and sapped of emotional energy.
Recognize that you are no longer who you used to be
and seek to resolve this crisis in your identity.

Recognize that you need a new identity to carry you into the future. Although a new identity won't erase the label you receive when you undergo a life transition, it will, when properly developed, provide new designations and status on a new smooth, paved road.

Power Tips

Be wise and do not take on too many things upon yourself during the period. Accept the limitations of your present situation

Manage your expectations. You may need to decrease the speed of your day-to-day operations till you get out of the muddy path of the transition.

PHASE 3

GETTING UNSTUCK

GETTING UNSTUCK

Unstuck! This is the phase you desire and should be in. As it is the solution phase to the initial problems you experience as a result of a life transition, it is a very important period. In fact, the process of getting unstuck is at the real heart of your life transition. However, this phase does not just happen in an instant. Getting unstuck requires your significant input.

In the stuck phase, you were spurred on to reflect on your situation, your environment, and your identity. You were encouraged to express your feelings and come to terms with your current situation. In the getting unstuck phase you will use what you discovered to get rid of the inertia that the change has caused.

The phase of getting unstuck requires action on your part, action that will get that stuck truck out of the muddy track and onto a better part of the track. The getting unstuck phase is when you remove those barriers that are holding you down on the spot. It is when you are liberated from the sticky mud and can plan the action steps you need to take to move forward.

The getting unstuck phase can be challenging because it requires great input from your side. You need your whole self—your mental capacity, your emotions, and a high level of awareness—for this phase. However, the results will be worth your effort in all respects. If you don't get unstuck, you will remain in the same spot. If you don't get rid of the obstacles pinning you down, you will not be able to attain the freedom you require to continue your journey.

You should also know that much of the personal growth and development that result from a life transition occurs in this phase. The whole process of putting your best foot forward helps you mature as a person.

So what does it really take to get unstuck?

Chapter 5

HOW DO I GET UNSTUCK?

In the last three chapters you discovered a lot about your current situation, how you got into it, and who you are now as a result. Through a process of introspection and deep questioning, you gathered vital information on these three parameters. In the current chapter you will learn how to use the vital knowledge you have gleaned to get rid of the sticky factors holding you down.

Brian's Method for Getting his Truck Unstuck

After calming down and accepting that his truck is stuck in a muddy track, Brian begins to think quite clearly. After all, he is not a novice when it comes to motoring issues. He starts to recollect a few things he had learned in his young adult years. He wonders why he had let the whole situation throw him off balance. Maybe it was just the scary thought that the place was quite isolated and he was alone that had tripped him off.

Brian decides to list in his mind the possible steps he can take to get his truck out of the muddy track. He uses the information he gathered about the alignment of the wheels to figure out which direction he should steer to get the tires out of the track (away from the impression line created by the tires). If the tires are out of the deep path of the track, he will at least be able to move the truck away slightly and use other tricks to get it farther from the area of the muddy track. "I just need to move the truck a few feet," he reckons. "That will be a good starting point."

Just then, another vehicle comes out of nowhere. Before Brian can wave or take any other action to stop the car from entering the muddy area, the second vehicle plummets into the track, just behind Brian. "Oh no!" Brian cries. "I was trying to wave and warn him, but that did not work."

Now there are two stuck drivers in the muddy path. After much consultation with each other, Brian and the other driver decide to help each other get their vehicles out of the messy situation in which they have found themselves. Since Brian's truck is in front, the two drivers start pushing it first until they finally get it out of the muddy track.

How Long Does it Take to Get Unstuck?

In Chapter 3 I discussed the two contrary mindsets you can have about life transitions. I explained that you can either maintain the perspective that transitions are rude interruptions to your normal life or that they are avenues for growth.

It is very important to reiterate here that different life-changing events pose different levels of challenges to the individual. The challenges posed by the loss of a loved one differ tremendously from those posed by relocation to a new city. The challenges Savannah faces as a result of her divorce are quite different from those confronting Paul, the car salesman who lost his job. And, as mentioned in Chapter 4, the level of readjustment required after different life transitions varies significantly, as depicted by Thomas Holmes and Richard Rahe's Social Re-adjustment Rating Scale.[2]

In addition, other factors out of your control may influence the time it takes you to get unstuck. Recovering from a natural disaster, for instance, depends on many external factors. Therefore, it may be difficult to predict the length of time that victims require to readjust and get back on track with their lives. The point is that there are no fixed timelines for getting unstuck when you are in a life transition.

---

[2]Holmes and Rahe, "Social Re-adjustment Rating Scale."

However, there is one pertinent determinant of the outcome of a transition that *is* within your control: your attitude. Your attitude and mindset toward the transition will influence how long it will take you to get unstuck. If you view the transition as a rude interruption and keep to that attitude, it may take you longer to figure out the essential steps you need to take to get unstuck. However, if you view the change as an avenue for growth, you will be more willing to get rid of the sticky factors and enter a new smooth, paved road.

Facing your fears about the change is an essential, bold step in preparing for your new journey.

Face Your Fears about Change

When you are faced with a life transition and you have been able to discover where you are and who you are in your new situation, the mere thought of a new smooth, paved road that is different from the one you were originally traveling on can be scary. Unknown things, unknown people, and unknown situations arouse varying degrees of fear and anxiety. Having to learn new ways of doing things or doing things in a new environment draws you out of your comfort zone. You may feel burdened and that there is too much risk involved.

Fear is a state of mind, an emotional reaction that is usually based on assumptions. If you are to face your fears and destroy their roots, you first need to identify them and call them by name. You then need to question the assumptions on which the fears are based and offer affirmations that are contrary to those assumptions and that provide a positive outlook on your future. You then need to continue to affirm that positive view on a regular basis.

Recognize Your Fears and Call Them by Name

The different kinds of fear that may arise when you experience change include fear of:

- The unknown
- Failure

- Rejection
- Incompetency
- Insufficient resources
- Inadequate finances
- Lifestyle adjustments
- Losing control

Depending on the particular type of transition, some fears are more prevalent than others. Someone who loses her job will have fears about financial issues, as will someone going through retirement, although in a different kind of way. Someone who is relocating to a new city will have a compendium of fears about the new environment and issues such as finding schools for the kids, a new job for the trailing spouse, new friends, new associates, and so on.

It is essential to identify the exact types of fears you have concerning the change you have faced. Ask yourself:

- What are the monsters hiding under this bridge of transition?

Identifying your fears and calling them by name is the first step toward downgrading any hold they might have on you.

Annihilate Your Fears

When you recognize the fears you have about your life transition, ask yourself questions about the assumptions underlying those fears. For example, your fear may be that people in your new location will not like you. That is the voice of a saboteur. Instead, ask, "What if they actually like me?" That is a 180-degree shift of the situation. Take this contrary view as your new paradigm. Focus on the fact that people will in fact like you in your new location.

Carry out affirmations based on this positive view. Tell people that you are moving into an unfamiliar environment and that you believe people in the new place will like you.

By doing this you are essentially quashing the voice of the saboteur and enhancing the voice of your new paradigm.

Elena Enumerates Her Fears about Her Transition

Elena, the survivor of Hurricane Katrina, has a long list of fears she has to face. Her greatest fear is that she may never get her life back together again. After much thought, Elena realizes this is an overarching view of her whole situation. She decides to break down the issues at stake and identify her specific fears about the change.

She identifies fears about her new location of Chicago; a new business/career or means of earning an income; her extended family—the ones who survived the hurricane; and about her very faith and whether she will be able to revive her spiritual vigor.

Elena then attempts to break down these areas even further. For example, regarding her business/career, Elena fears that she might have to take an alternative job, that she will lack resources to start a new business, that she will be rejected in a new neighborhood even if she does succeed in opening a new diner, and that she'll never find the kind of capable staff she used to have. These are all very intimidating fears for Elena, and she has similarly daunting lists in the other areas.

She decides it is too stressful to consider all of these issues at once. It would be better to look at each stage as it arises. This decision is very uplifting to her. She decides to talk about her fears to those around her and take care of them stage by stage. As she talks to her new neighbors and employs the services of professionals, Elena begins to gradually affirm the positive view she needs to overcome the fear she faced at the initial stages of her huge transition.

Identify Factors That May Be Preventing You from Getting Unstuck

Once you have been able to create alternative paradigms to counteract your fear and you have started affirming this new view, you will have some mental space to do some analysis. This is the opportunity to take an objective look at your muddy path in order to identify the factors keeping you in the stuck position.

Ask yourself:

- What are the sticky factors holding me down in this muddy path?
- In what way(s) are they holding me down?
- What is preventing me from getting unstuck?

The answers to these questions will help you delineate the actions you need to carry out to get unstuck. For instance, if Brian the stuck truck driver identifies that one of his tires is in the center of a pothole, his approach for getting it out may involve lifting and hauling. However, if the situation is that a tire is blocked by a rock, he may need to twist the steering wheel to one side or the other to get the car unstuck.

Get Rid of the Sticky Factors

You might expect that you will quickly be able to get rid of the factors keeping you in a stuck position once you have identified what they are. But identifying the sticky factors is only one step toward eliminating them.

Shift your mindset

The pivotal step to clear away the obstacles in your path is to shift your mindset. This requires you to look at your situation with a contrary view. A simple example is viewing something you feel is impossible as actually very possible.

In a bid to take an alternative view, look at how you perceived your current situation at the onset of the change. Your initial perceptions were discussed in Chapter 2. That chapter used several metaphors to help you express how you were feeling at that point. Reframing the metaphor that describes how you felt could help you develop an alternative view of your situation. This in turn will help shift your mindset to one that guides you to a new smooth, paved road.

For example, if you felt or still feel overpowered or overwhelmed, then probe and ask:

- What is the power holding me down?

Once you are able to delineate what or who this power is, take time to offer yourself a 180-degree shift in your views about this powerful object. See it as a power that is not going to hold you down any longer. Downgrade the level this power has in your mind's eye.

Do you feel trapped in or hedged in? Then ask:

- What is holding me prisoner?

Do you feel pinned down? Then probe:

- What is holding me down?

Do you feel stuck in the middle of nowhere? Then ask:

- In what way am I both tied down and detached?

Viewing your situation from a pose that is contrary to the one you had at the onset of the change will help prepare you for the actions you need to take to remove the obstacles. With a shift in your perceptions, most things that seemed impossible suddenly become possible. That is why this mindset shift is very critical. It can be compared to the push that Brian gave his truck to get it off the muddy path. It is a big push and a mighty haul that will position you for success in the future.

Things you need to stop doing to further establish your freedom

1. Stop putting too much blame on the cause of the transition or the events that led to it. As discussed in Chapter 3, when you have identified the cause of your transition, take time to talk about it and grieve. However, do not do this as a way of re-victimizing yourself. You need to move forward. Instead of spending your energy on maintaining the stimulus event in your mind, downgrade it and create more mental space. You need that space to find means of getting unstuck.

2. Stop wallowing in self-pity.

3. Stop striving for what you had in the past.

Things you need to start doing to reinforce your freedom

1. Permit yourself to get rid of any identity factors that are no longer serving you. It could be that they served you well in the past, but you now need to start on a new, paved road.

2. Affirm that you are making a shift. Affirm that you are actually going to start something new.

3. Tell others about your intentions to seek a new smooth, paved road.

4. Continue to resolve the crisis you may still be feeling about your lost identity by taking more appropriate steps to mourn and say goodbye to it (as discussed in Chapter 4).

Which sticky factors are you not willing to let go of?

Having let go of some of the sticky factors you identified, you may find that, for some reason, you are holding on to a few. Maybe you found it easy to get rid of some but that others are too sacred to let go of, and therefore you have left them intact.

If you carry out only a partial elimination of sticky factors you will have only limited success in your attempt to move on. After a few steps forward you will probably find yourself being pulled backward by factors that you left untouched. That is why it is necessary to perform another check after an appropriate period to ensure that you have indeed let go of all the sticky factors.

Ask yourself:

- Which of these sticky factors am I not willing to let go of?
- Which aspects of the muddy path am I protecting?

If you are holding on to a sticky factor because you feel it is too sacred to let go of, it could be that you have not mourned the aspect of your loss represented by that sticky factor. Take time to mourn adequately. Do what it takes to say goodbye physically. For instance, if you need to travel to a place to do a private memorial for an item or issue, invest some time and energy to do it. Then say goodbye and leave it there.

It could be that the sticky factor itself is an effect that you desire in something, a sense of fulfillment that something you have lost once provided. You may find it hard to let that effect go as it actually contributes to your well-being. In such cases, you could find alternative ways of getting that effect. For example, a newly retired person may find it hard to let go of a certain aspect of work-derived fulfillment that made him feel worthy. Finding an alternative means of getting that type of work-derived fulfillment (such as by mentoring others) will help this person let go of the stickiness of the past.

As you acquire the wisdom to get rid of the tough sticky factors, you will gain the power you need for moving on fully.

Diane Offers a Contrary View to the Voice of the Saboteur

For Diane, the woman diagnosed with lupus, going through a mindset shift is challenging. She finds it hard to envision how she will be able to enjoy her life on a new smooth road that is different from the one on which she had good health. After much effort, Diane is able to answer the question, "What is overpowering me?" When she probes honestly, she finds that her greatest fear is that she won't be able to run her business as she had before her illness. The contrary view is that there is a way out of this situation, even if Diane can't see it yet. She realizes she has to maintain that contrary view if she is to have enough mental space to find any alternative solutions. Diane therefore resolves to downgrade the fear in her mind. She then affirms that there is a way onto a new smooth, paved road, and that she is ready to do some exploration in this regard.

Enlist Resources for Getting Rid of the Sticky Factors

If Brian's truck had been so badly stuck that he needed more resources to get it out of the muddy path, he would have had to call on some outside body for help. Apart from the help he had received from the driver of the other vehicle that came by, Brian might have needed the services of a tow truck.

It is possible that you may not have enough resources at hand to get unstuck all by yourself. In such a case, it is wise to seek external help to get rid of the obstacles.

Professional coaches—life coaches, career coaches, and/or business coaches—can help you delineate means of getting unstuck during a life transition. They can help you through the initial process of getting rid of sticky factors. They can support you in mapping alternative perspectives that will work in your new situation. They can be your accountability partners as you draw out new goals and action plans for moving forward in your new situation.

Note that coaching professionals are better able to help you when you are actually ready to get unstuck and move forward. If you are still in the process of grieving your loss or you require more time to mourn, you are best matched with a counselor equipped to help you heal through therapy work based on your history.

In this chapter I have highlighted the importance of identifying and then getting rid of the factors keeping you in a stuck position. I discussed how you need to face your fears about the change and how a mindset shift can help you believe in your ability to enter a new smooth, paved road. This shift can create the awareness you need to assume an "I can" pose.

Having rid yourself of the sticky factors and having prepared your mind to explore, the question that now comes to mind is, "Where do I go now?" This topic is the subject of the next chapter.

Wisdom Tips

Face your fears about the future. Do not let them paralyze you physically and emotionally. Question the assumptions on which the fears are based and offer affirmations that are contrary to those assumptions and that provide a positive outlook on your future.

Re-ignite your passion by taking on new avenues for fulfillment. Re-assure yourself that as you take time to substitute new things, new involvement into your routine, you will find alternative means of getting the fulfillment that doing the issue that you can no longer do used to give you.

Power Tips

Stop wallowing in self-pity. Stop striving for what you had in the past. That tends to be a waste of energy especially if it is linked to an identity that no longer exists.

Partial elimination of sticky factors that are holding you down will result only in limited success in your attempt to move on. You need to get rid of all of them. As you acquire the wisdom to get rid of the tough sticky factors, you will gain the power you need for moving on fully.

PHASE 4

MOVING ON

MOVING ON

Moving on—how exciting! After all, what is the use of getting unstuck if you are going to stay in the area of the muddy path from which you have just been liberated? That would not be so fruitful. No, the real reason you sought to get unstuck is so you can move on and continue your journey on a new smooth, paved road. The excitement and sense of freedom you experienced when you got unstuck should now be directed toward creating a new path that will work for your onward journey.

Having experienced enormous growth and development during the process of getting unstuck, you now have a foundation to build upon as you tackle the moving-on phase. This period is about finding opportunities to create new memories on a new smooth, paved road. It is about seeking new pathways to fulfillment in your modified circumstances. As a result, the moving-on phase is quite inviting. Nevertheless, like other phases of transition, it has its challenges. The fact that you are heading into an unknown zone means you have to take some risks. Apart from this you need to replenish your sanity and strength, because you have spent a lot of these resources on getting unstuck.

Finding new power requires you to release a lot of emotional garbage and go through a further mindset shift. However, doing this will position you for more growth and development, which will in turn prepare you to take on more challenges that you might face during this phase. But be assured: the challenges are worth taking on and there is light at the end of the tunnel.

So what does it take to move on? How do you enter a new smooth, paved road in your life's journey?

Chapter 6

WHERE DO I GO NOW?

In the previous chapter I discussed the pivotal step of getting unstuck from the muddy pathway by getting rid of the sticky factors holding you down. I also highlighted how this crucial step was only the beginning of your reentry onto a smooth, paved road. However, to be fully able to enter and take ownership of that new smooth, paved road, you need to take some solid steps to kick off the motion. This motion-initiating stage typically begins with your taking time to delineate the direction of your reentry journey. It starts with an exploration of your options in the new circumstances that the change has created. This process is the focus of the current chapter.

Brian the Truck Driver Takes Stock

When Brian finally liberates his truck from the muddy track, it is not only his truck that gets unstuck. Brian himself feels as if a heavy load has been lifted from his shoulders. Oh, what a relief! He thanks the driver of the other vehicle profusely for his help. Then the two of them work together to get the second vehicle out of the muddy track. This vehicle is a lot easier to get moving again since its sticky track was not as deep as for Brian's truck.

With both vehicles out, Brian relishes his freedom for some time. But then a question comes to his mind: "Where do I go now?" As he had discovered right after getting stuck, the muddy track was not headed in the exact direction he had originally been traveling. His truck had been diverted. Fortunately, Brian had figured out his bearings shortly after getting stuck. However, the question still remains: "Where am I to go now?"

A number of options occur to him. He can find a means of getting back to the route he was taking before the diversion. Alternatively, he can explore a totally new route that will still take him to where he was going before he got stuck. A third option is to take a new route to an entirely new destination. He decides to take some time to weigh each of these options before making a final decision.

Take Stock of Where You Were Going before You Got Stuck

Before Brian can decide which option to take to resume his journey, he realizes that he has to bring his original intention into sharp focus. "Where was I going before I got stuck?" he asks himself. He knows he has to retrace the route back to his original smooth, paved road in order to pursue the first option. If, on the other hand, he takes the second option to create a new route altogether, he still needs to know where he was going. And if he decides that, because of his recent experience, there is no longer any need to go where he was originally headed, he still needs to figure out where he should go now that he is free.

Like Brian, you need to take stock to decide on the direction of your next move. This involves taking a critical look at your life before the change occurred. Take a retrospective look at where you were heading before you were diverted. Then take an introspective look and ask yourself what your original purposes were in life. What were your dreams? What did you want to achieve down the road before you entered the muddy path?

De-clutter Your Mental and Physical Spaces

To see clearly enough to answer these questions, it may be necessary for you to de-clutter both your physical and mental spaces. Remove any physical items that may prevent you from seeing clearly. If there are items that you have said mental goodbyes to but are still keeping, move them out of your range of vision. Once you clear the clutter it will be easier to see what is essential to your new life direction.

You also need to de-clutter your mental space. Stop wallowing in self-pity. This process of looking at your past goals is meant to identify what you need to take forward in terms of previous dreams and lessons learned.

Once you are able to achieve clarity you will be able to analyze your previous goals and sort them into categories such as:

- Dump altogether
- Keep as is
- Modify to fit new circumstances

The goals you file under the "keep as is" and "modify to fit new circumstances" categories are the ones you need to take forward as you proceed with your journey.

Take a Fresh Look at Your Life's Purpose

In Chapter 1 I explained how we as human beings pass through phases of emotional crisis either in mid-life or at other times when we question our existential values. Periods of transition in general make us question the real meaning of our existence—why we are here on this earth at this moment in time. We probe the very purpose of our lives. This kind of questioning is very essential for us to make some meaning out of what has happened. We need to ask these questions to put things more into focus, especially during the phase when we are making decisions about which path to take in our forward journey.

So, after taking stock of the intentions, dreams, and plans you had before you got stuck in the muddy path, it is very helpful to take a fresh look at your life's purpose, the reason why you are here on Earth. Simply put, discovering your purpose is like figuring out what you want to do with the rest of your life. It is about what you will be striving for on that new smooth, paved road. With a purpose for continuing on, you will be more motivated to tackle challenges you might find on your way because you have something to strive for.

If you don't identify your purpose for existence, even minor challenges may seem too difficult and you may tend to give in and fall out before achieving your target goals. Delineating your life's purpose puts you in a position where you are more resolute and, therefore, more likely to make it through to a new you.

To find your life's purpose, take time to answer the following questions in a relaxed atmosphere:

- What do I love doing?
- What do I enjoy doing so much that I lose track of time?
- What do I do so effortlessly and naturally that it seems like breathing to me?
- What have I done in the past that made me feel great?
- What was I doing when I felt a great sense of fulfillment or accomplishment?

Answering these questions will help you draw out what your purpose is and when you have felt "on purpose." From these answers try to carve out a statement that describes your purpose. The following are examples of purpose statements:

"My purpose is to be like water to my family—
refreshing, cleansing, and purifying."

"My purpose is to become an accomplished
guitarist."

"My purpose is to radiate the goodness of God
to others."

"My purpose is to be a linchpin that connects
this generation and the next."

Keep your purpose statement in a place where you can see it frequently.

Knowing your life's purpose is not the end in itself. Once you have clearly stated your purpose you need to use it as the lens through which you make decisions about your new journey. Focusing on your life's purpose will help you analyze more objectively the various options you have for entering a new smooth, paved road.

Savannah Has to Explore
Her Options in Many Areas of Her Life

Savannah decides to explore the options available to her in her new status as a divorced woman. First, it seems to her that she needs to be firm in her mind that her role has changed in the family setting. She recognizes this acknowledgement is at the core of any new decisions. It is at the heart of her ability to acquire the sanity and strength required at this phase of her life.

After this reinforced acknowledgement, Savannah is able to affirm that she needs a new direction for her life—one that may be quite different from her original intentions.

With the divorce and her change in status, Savannah first needs to redefine many aspects of day-to-day living. To work out her life without Fred, she needs significant mental capacity. The core of the change is that there is no Fred to share her whole life with. No Fred to share her dreams and aspirations with. No Fred to unwind together with after work. No family time with Fred and the children at the beach on sunny days.

One of the most important issues at stake is how she will raise the children all by herself. The new arrangement is that Fred will have them over at his new place on alternative weekends. His new place? That also is a strange concept. "How will I keep up with what used to be our house, our finances, our chores, our duties, and so on, all by myself?" she wonders. That will definitely demand a change in the way things used to operate.

She then asks herself another question: "Do I still want to keep going in the same direction?" She thinks about how difficult that will be in many areas of her life. As she ponders the babysitting arrangements, the housekeeping, the kids' schooling, and other issues, Savannah realizes that she needs to modify many aspects of her journey to fit her new circumstances, especially with respect to raising her kids.

Savannah then considers the issue of her current employment. Can she afford to stay on at a job that requires a fair amount of travel while raising two young children on her own? This is a big and important issue to resolve. Savannah knows she might have to consider an alternative route for her career. However, before re-launching her life after the huge change she has experienced, she knows she should take some time to analyze her options before making decisions that will affect her long-term success.

Analyze Your Options and
Make Informed Decisions

To make informed decisions about the direction in which to resume your forward journey, you need to research the different options you identified in your discovery process. Just like Brian the truck driver chose to do, it is wise to get as much information as you can about what the rest of your journey would look like if you were to take your original intended route. Ask yourself the questions:

- Is the road ahead clearer than where I am?
- Will I still encounter more mud pits along the way?
- Is it safe to continue on this route or is it better to find another route altogether?

The answers to these questions will help you make a basic decision on whether or not to continue on the same route to the same destination as before you were diverted by a life transition. You can then use this foundational knowledge to determine what other options you may need to research, such as new destinations and/or new routes.

Since the change event you have experienced has likely impacted different areas of your life and identity (see Chapter 4), take time to research the options available to you in the areas of career, finances, health and physical fitness, spirituality, and others. Your research should take into account which combinations of the options you discover will work best together in your new situation.

For instance, someone experiencing a health-related life transition should research health care options to move toward a cure and/or better quality of life. If this individual was also a significant income earner for her family but is unable to continue in her previous job because of her health issues, she also needs to research new options for generating income. She may also want to research available fitness options that will work in synergy with her medical treatments or that will help her maintain an acceptable quality of life despite her health condition.

Paul Revisits His Original Career Dreams

During his stock-taking exercise, Paul rediscovers what his original career goal had been before he became a car salesman. He had originally dreamed about going to college and taking a professional course. Now, with his job at the car dealership gone and his wife's job hours cut back, Paul decides to research the options available to him at this crossroads in his life.

With a family of three kids, the oldest in his tweens, Paul knows he has many issues at stake. He feels pressured to make the right decisions for his family to survive. At the same time, Paul knows he should not yield to these pressures and make a hurried decision. Although he may have to make some choices immediately, he decides to see them as temporary decisions while he researches his options thoroughly for more permanent solutions.

Paul goes to the local library to review a copy of *Career Connections*. Paul also remembers one additional tool he has that could be very useful at this phase of his life: his personal rolodex. Over the course of his employment at the car dealership he had met a wide range of people and he had been diligent about putting the business cards he had collected in this rolodex. Paul pulls it out and puts his networking back into full gear.

While doing all this research related to employment and careers, Paul realizes he also has to obtain more information regarding his wife's hip surgery. He has to look for information on rehabilitation after the surgery and the options available for her to continue work at the TV station, perhaps in a different department. He has lots to look into, but Paul feels confident there are ways forward.

Map Your Journey to Fit Your New Circumstances

Based on your stock-taking exercise, you may have been able to refocus on your original intentions, especially in the area of your transition. You now need to create a new set of goals to bridge the gap between where you are now and the future life you have envisioned.

Take time to think critically about the question:

- Do I still want to keep going in the same direction?

Depending on your answer, you may either want to try to find your way back to your original route or to find a new route altogether.

Charting a new course for your journey on the original route

If your answer to the question above is an objective "yes," then you may need to re-strategize how to get to your desired place following the same route you were taking before. To do this, you may need to modify many aspects of your journey to fit your current situation. Modification may mean a new sequence to the events in the journey, an addition to the existing plan, or a new method or vehicle for getting to one or more points during the journey. Your modification strategy should take into account what you are now able to do and the resources you currently have, as opposed to what you could do or what you had in your old situation.

Mapping out an altogether new route for your journey

If your answer to the question above is a resounding "no," you will need to create a plan that will take you through an altogether different route.

After Brian the truck driver retraces the route between where he was and where he got stuck, he goes further and analyzes the original purpose for the journey he was on. It is then that he recognizes that it is no use to try to get back on the original route he was traveling before he got diverted. Having reexamined his journey's purpose, he concludes that the previous route will not get him to where he wants to go. Brian resolves that the best way out is to draw a new plan via an alternative route.

In your particular situation, it may be that when you took stock and revisited your life's purpose, you decided that it is no longer worthwhile to go to where you were headed before. Perhaps your previous goals will not help you accomplish your new life mission. In this case, you may need to dump those previous goals. You need to be flexible and have an open mind to delineate new goals that will help you fulfill your new mission.

We human beings tend to prefer the familiar—the old route— rather than a new path that will require extra effort to map out. However, taking the time to outline new goals will work to your advantage. If you have realized that you need to map out a totally different route, take courage and go for this choice. It is better to begin anew than to try to patch up something that may not work in your new circumstances.

In addition, taking shortcuts to your new route in order to avoid having to start fresh may end up being a total waste of your precious time and energy. While shortcuts may seem appealing and easy, they can be dangerous and energy-sapping. They tend to be slippery, causing you to fall each time you attempt to walk on them. Instead, focus on mapping out a proper route that will land you on a new smooth, paved road.

Ask:

- What are the possibilities here?
- What new options can I create?

In the preceding discussion on analyzing options, I stated that you should find the right combination of options that will work in your situation. At times, such a combination does not exist, at least not in your locality. Part of mapping out an altogether new route for your journey involves creating that option combination yourself. This creative process can open the door to great possibilities in the future.

Prepare for the Journey Ahead

With a new or modified route in hand, you are partly equipped to resume your journey. Before you head for the start line, however, you need a few other items: a new sense of direction and a new identity. You may need to acquire other things once you get going, but these are highly essential at the outset.

Finding a new sense of direction

As discussed in Chapter 2, the change you initially experienced left you in a confused state. However, when you worked on getting the confusion out, you came to recognize where you are in your current situation. To move forward from that spot after getting unstuck, you need to have a new sense of direction. You need to reset your internal compass so you know which direction leads to the west, for instance. This will help you move from a disoriented state to an oriented one.

You can also hone a new sense of direction by envisioning the future in the new destination you have chosen. What does life look like there? This thought is empowering and will boost your self-confidence.

Continue to combat your fears about the journey ahead. Stick with the affirmations you started. Continue to believe that you are fully capable of going through the transition. Affirm your ability to find new fulfillment on a new smooth, paved road.

Searching for a new identity

In Chapter 4 I guided you through the process of envisioning yourself in the future without the identity you have lost. That process must have made you realize there is a gap that needs to be filled. Since you cannot function properly in the future without an identity, you need to search for a new one—just like Savannah, who can no longer use her lost identity as Fred's wife. She needs to seek a new identity that is not linked to this role or status. You have a similar challenge.

So, based on the future you have envisioned, start searching. Start seeking a new identity, one that is not directly linked to the role or status you had before your life transition. This new identity will be pivotal to the success of your newly resumed journey.

Doug Manning refers to the struggle with identity after bereavement in his book, *Don't Take My Grief Away From Me*.[3] He states: "You must forge a new identity in the midst of all of the pressures of grief and the struggle for appropriate behavior... It is almost like being eighteen years of age again and struggling to find yourself. A great deal of time must be spent in sorting through feelings to discover how you feel about life... and evaluating your worth."

With an open mind, take time to explore what kind of things you could be doing in the areas of your career, your family, your hobby, and so on, that will give you a new sense of self—a new sense of who you are.

---

[3]Doug Manning, Don't Take My Grief Away From Me (San Francisco: HarperOne, 1984), 104.

One Size May Not Fit All When Many People Are Involved

Some transitions are so complex that you may need to make more than one attempt to delineate where you want to go. This is the case in relationship-based transitions that affect not only you but a number of other people.

For example, for someone who has experienced the loss of a family member, decisions about the new direction should take into account the needs of all the other family members. Some of these needs may collide while the family is trying to find the new direction. This will require multiple attempts at drawing and redrawing new directions. If you are in this situation, take heart: none of these attempts is a wasted process. Instead, they all add up in the healing journey and a significant amount of growth can take place if you keep a positive attitude. Have an open mind and continue to acquire the sanity and strength to draw out these directions.

Challenge the Status Quo

At times, the drawing out of a new route may require you to challenge the status quo. You may need to challenge the norms and current beliefs of the society in which you live or the unwritten rules of workplace culture and career practices. On the other hand, you may need to challenge family traditions that limit what you can do or achieve. When you take a critical look, you may even find that such beliefs are among the sticky factors that kept you stuck in the first place.

For example, a middle-aged woman had always wished she could work in a certain industry but was restricted by her family, which followed an unwritten rule that working in such an industry would violate their family tradition. When this woman lost the job she had, which conformed with this belief, she decided to challenge the family restriction and map out a new direction for her career based on what she had always wished for.

To challenge the status quo of tradition or cultural beliefs, you need to think outside the lines that might have been drawn by such beliefs or tradition. Take a stab at the status quo. Offer a contrary view and continue to affirm it. Take your stand to defend it. Make it real by setting it as your new direction.

In this chapter I have elaborated on how to explore your options as you consider where to go after getting liberated from factors that previously held you stuck. When you analyze each of the options you discover, you need to view them through the lens of your newly refocused life's purpose. When you decide on which option(s) to pursue, you will be moving closer to re-launching your journey.

So how do you get to that new place of your choice? This is the subject of the next chapter.

Wisdom Tips

Discovering and developing a new sense of self and identity in all areas of your life is a gateway to success in your new circumstances.

Re-discovering your purpose after you get unstuck is like figuring out what you want to do with the rest of your life. It is about what you will be striving for on your new smooth, paved road.

Power Tips

When you release emotional garbage from the past, you will find new power to take on more challenges that may occur as you move on.

Stop seeking 'short-cut' routes to your new destination. Even though appealing, such could be dangerous and energy-sapping. Instead, focus on mapping out new strategies that will land you on a new solid path.

Chapter 7

HOW DO I GET TO THAT NEW PLACE?

In the last chapter I discussed ways of deciphering which direction to take to move forward in your life's journey once you get unstuck. I explained the concepts of analyzing your options and mapping your route as the basis of setting off anew in the direction you have chosen.

You now need to set new goals to achieve those dream destinations you have identified on your new journey map. This chapter equips you for moving from exploration to action. It discusses how to break down your journey into milestones that you can set goals toward achieving. It elaborates on how to discover a new identity with which to move forward and how to get the power you require to execute the action steps to achieve your goals.

Brian the Truck Driver Decides to Use an Alternative Route

Brian the truck driver finally decides which of the options he is going to take to resume his journey. He chooses an alternative route from the one he had originally been traveling on before the diversion. This requires a totally different plan from the one he had before. However, Brian is resolved that this is the way out, especially when he realizes there are more muddy potholes on the road he has been diverted onto. The forecast of the journey on this road is not so good.

Brian also realizes it is no use trying to get back on to his original road. That road would lead him to a destination he no longer desires now that he has brought the purpose of his journey back into focus after getting unstuck.

Given all of this, Brian decides to map out a new course of action. He decides to set goals for the new journey ahead. He then breaks those goals down into small steps.

Just like Brian, you need to set new goals for the route you have chosen to resume your journey. Getting to that new place requires a bridge that connects the old situation with the new. And setting goals is like designing actions for crossing that bridge.

Set SMART Goals

To be the most effective, the goals you set for your new journey should be SMART, which is an acronym for:

Specific—defined, unambiguous

Measurable—can be quantified or assessed

Attainable—may be a stretch but is achievable

Relevant—aligned with your purpose

Time-sensitive—can be accomplished within a specific time

SMART goals lend themselves to accountability and, therefore, increase your chances of success. Find an accountability partner who can support you in the execution of the action steps toward your goals. It is also helpful to use the support of discerning companions or members of a community group who are addressing a similar transition.

Define What "Momentum" Means to You at This Phase

The SMART acronym has the letters "A" for attainable and "T" for time-sensitive. Since you have just experienced change, some of the goals you are setting out to accomplish may take longer to achieve than when you were previously on the smooth, paved road. This is especially true at the initial stage of moving on.

Give yourself time to readjust. In this regard, recognize that you are the one to define what "momentum" means at each particular phase of the transition. Recognize that the more you move forward, even if it is at a slow pace at the beginning, the better off you'll be. With each step you take you are moving away from the stuck position and making progress. With each step you will also be learning and better positioned for success than if you had remained in the same place after getting unstuck.

Ryan Sets Goals for a New Career Action Plan

Ryan, the computer associate who suffered a terrible injury in a workplace accident, has analyzed his options for moving forward. Since the accident left him bound to a wheelchair, he has to figure out what to do regarding his career. The medical personnel working with him have been very informative and supportive about mobility and related issues, and he has been addressing the issue of his relationship with the girl he had been seeing. But the huge thing on Ryan's mind is his career. His time of service at the local start-up firm had been very short and he was still on probationary part-time employment at the time of the accident. As stated in his terms of services with the company, he is not yet entitled to any benefits.

After considerable thought, Ryan decides to establish a consulting business. He feels he will have a more fulfilled life doing something he really loves, and computing is his passion. Ryan breaks down this big goal into smaller ones, such as researching information about starting a consulting business, taking online courses to brush up his skills as necessary, researching the market to find out what aspects of computing are hot and relevant, and obtaining funding to start a company. He then takes each of these goals and outlines action steps for achieving them. Ryan sets target dates for achieving his goals so he can prod himself on for success.

Discover a New Identity

In Chapter 4 I discussed how you needed to search for a new identity since the one you had before the change is lost and gone forever. And in Chapter 6 I discussed the importance of finding your life's purpose. Your newly discovered purpose is an important tool in many aspects of moving forward. In particular, your purpose will be of tremendous help in your discovery of a new identity as you pursue your journey on a new smooth, paved road.

Your total identity is made up of how you present yourself in various areas of your life. That means your search for a new identity should encompass carving out new identities in each of the following areas.

A new sense of self through a boost of your self-esteem

Your sense of self and your self-esteem are intricately linked. If you feel you are worthy and that your day-to-day activities are meaningful, this will tend to boost your self-esteem. If you are part of a community where you have a sense of belonging, loneliness will decrease because you feel needed and that your presence (and, therefore, your existence) is meaningful.

You will discover a new sense of self as you find means of replacing or restoring the sense of fulfillment you derived from something you lost in the transition. For instance, if you are recently retired, try and find some means of maintaining your job-derived fulfillment. This could be mentoring other professionals or serving on a board of an organization whose mandate is in your area of expertise or passion. These kinds of activities will boost your self-esteem and, thus, your sense of self.

For different types of transitions, increased self-esteem may develop as you take on:

- New opportunities, such as mentoring or volunteering
- New ways of nurturing yourself, such as a mini-vacation, food, music, or recreation
- New avenues for creative expression, such as art, writing, or photography
- New behavior patterns

A new social/community identity

Depending on the life-changing event that has occurred, you might try some of the following to form a new social/community identity:

- Engage in new work-related associations (if you have lost a job or career)
- Find new avenues for making a circle of friends
- Join clubs, recreation centers, and hobby groups
- Revive past friendships (for example, if you have lost a spouse and most of your friendships were jointly made, continue to tap into those friendships in new ways as a single person)

A new family identity

If you have lost a spouse or family member, a new family identity will form as you:

- Establish a new relationship with your loved one through memory

- Finish a project started by your spouse/family member
- Support the cause he/she fought for
- Create an album in his/her memory
- Redefine the roles played by different members of your family to conform with your new status
- Use the supportive structure of in-laws and extended family
- Pay a visit to the place of your roots

A new economic identity

For many life-changing events, a new economic identity is required to move on. You can adjust to your new economic status by trying to:

- Balance your new lifestyle with your new income status by making new choices regarding:
- Where you live
- Where you shop
- The type of car you drive
- The type of key amenities you purchase
- Your major expenses
- Make use of support from community resources

A new spiritual identity

A great part of your identity comes from expression of your spirituality. You may discover a new spiritual identity as you:

- Join a faith community
- Tap into available resources that help you connect with God
- Spend time alone in nature

- Explore the object of your loved one's spirituality and/or belief (if you have lost a close relationship)

- Seek a well-grounded spiritual person to whom you can pose questions

A new career or intellectual identity

This is especially relevant if you have lost a job or are experiencing a career-related transition, including due to family relocation or a health challenge that prevents you from performing your previous job. A new career or intellectual identity takes shape as you:

- Tap into available resources for procuring a new job

- Network through all available means

- If necessary, take extra education to upgrade your skills

- Are open to jobs of a different nature

- Are ready to use your transferable skills

As you work on all of these different areas of your identity, recognize that discovery is a continuous process and that it takes varying amounts of time. Recognize that you may feel overwhelmed at times. Do not try to do this all at once. It may be necessary to focus on your greatest area of need first. Learn to go at your own pace, but keep at it. Though it requires a great effort on your part, it is a worthwhile effort because it is a stepping stone to a new you.

Harry Creates a Digital Album in Memory of His Wife

Harry's late wife, Debra, who passed away forty years into their marriage, had a flair for international cuisine. She had always enjoyed foods from different parts of the world, and she had taken this passion to another level when she started the local International Cuisine Fair six years before her death. The popularity of the annual fair had grown tremendously over those six years.

As Harry tries hard to find a new identity for moving forward after Debra's death, he decides to create a digital album of memories about her. He decides that pulling together all the pictures and memorabilia of the Cuisine Fair is a good place to start.

Harry gathers the principal photographs taken at the event over the past six years. He then collects all the newspaper articles about the event. He has a few of the relevant newspaper issues at home, but he has to go to the local library to dig out the majority of the issues. It takes Harry some time to put the album together, but when it is all done he feels great about it.

In fact, the project boosts his self-esteem in many ways. Working on the album stimulates both his creative and intellectual sides. As a recent retiree, Harry also finds some work-derived fulfillment. Harry is of the old school, adding multimedia skills to his expertise only later in his work life. Therefore, going digital with the album project is a great boost to his self-esteem. Apart from the work aspect, doing the project also helps him reconnect with his and Debra's group of friends in a new way. When Harry shares the digital album with his three children, they are all very proud of what he has done in memory of their mom. It brings them even closer as a family.

Through this unique extension of the work that his late wife was fond of, Harry is able to not only honor his late wife's memory but also enjoy a new avenue for his own creative expression. In addition, his work on the project helps him find new means of social interaction, find a new sense of self, and build a new connection with his and Debra's three children. Harry is able to discover new identity parameters that can gradually help in his process of moving forward after his bereavement. It will take more time, but he has at least started regaining some motion through these unique small steps.

Acquire the Power to Move On

As mentioned in preceding sections on setting goals and discovering a new identity, the process of moving on requires a lot of input from your side. But at times you may feel that you do not have enough strength to tackle all that is required at this stage. How do you get this kind of strength on a day-to-day basis? How do you get the power to move on as you desire? Here are some tips to help you acquire such power.

Forgive and release the past

At times, the weariness you experience in the moving-on phase may be due to the fact that you have not forgiven the past. When you refuse to forgive the past, whether a particular incident or a particular set of people, you are giving your power away to bitterness, anger, and many other negative emotions. So ask yourself:

- To whom or to what circumstances have I given my power away through unforgiveness?

Forgive elements of the past that you feel had anything to do with your transition. Forgive yourself if you made any errors. Forgive the circumstances. Release those people and/or situations and get your power back.

Give yourself permission to do what is necessary to move on

Part of releasing the past may actually have to do with your attitude toward yourself. Do not hold onto the notion that you need to punish yourself for an error you may have made. That notion is not healthy. Similarly, if the transition was caused by something you had no control over, do not chastise yourself over it. For instance, if you have lost a spouse, you do not need to chastise yourself by withholding from joining social circles.

So ask yourself:

- What should I give myself permission to do in this phase of my transition?

- What should I give myself permission to do in order to move on?

Then go on and give yourself permission to do those things.

Reactivate areas of your life that were made stagnant by the change

Giving yourself permission to do what it takes to move on is a prodding step toward reactivating areas of your life made stagnant by the life transition. Ask:

- Which areas of my life have been made stagnant by the change?

- Which of these areas do I need to reactivate or plug back into the power source?

These areas could be such things as your relationships with members of your family, your work colleagues, or your boss. Or maybe the stagnant areas involve your physical fitness, general grooming, spirituality, intellectual pursuits, or family responsibilities. As you identify these areas, start working on revitalizing them with your newly discovered identity. Doing this will recharge your life's batteries, which were run down by the life transition. As you gradually reignite your passion for life, your power to move on will come more naturally.

Laugh

Laugh at yourself. Use laughter to lessen the stress of your situation or problem. When you laugh at yourself and your problems, you are able to deal with that pain in a focused but lighter fashion, putting you in a better position to move through the situation causing the pain and, ultimately, get beyond it.

Abraham Lincoln said: "With the fearful strain that is on me night and day, if I did not laugh I should die."

Maintain your physical and mental well-being

Take time to do what it takes to keep physically fit. Go to the gym. Participate in various sporting activities. Keeping physically fit will help give you the reserves of energy you need at this phase. In addition, you should eat well and nourish your body in as many ways as possible. Pay attention to your mental well-being.

Make Use of Power Tools

To get to that new place you dream of, you will also benefit from the support of discerning companions and professionals. I call these your power tools.

Use the support of discerning companions and mentors

When you resume your journey it is helpful to enlist the support of a group of people as you execute your new action steps. This group of people could include friends, family members, or leaders in your community. Individually and/or collectively, these people can provide physical and mental support to you as you wade your way through unfamiliar territories. The moral support of a listening ear offered by a discerning companion can be of great help in maintaining your sanity and strength throughout the moving-on phase. You may also enlist the support of mentors, who could be leaders or ordinary people whose firm belief in you will reassure you that you can make it through to the next goal in your plan.

Use professional support

In Chapter 4 I mentioned the role that professional coaches can play in supporting you through the process of transition. When you are ready to enter the action phase in pursuit of your new goals, coaches can serve as your accountability partners and help keep you on track as you gather momentum in your new journey. As necessary, they can also help you refocus on your goals should you get sidetracked.

Face Your Fears about Moving On

In Chapter 5 I discussed the issue of facing your fears about the change you are going through. After you have gotten unstuck and have begun to map out the route to a new smooth, paved road, you might experience more periods of fear and anxiety as the reality of what it will take to get that new place dawns on you. You might have been able to assess the risks involved more objectively, but now that it's time for action, it is possible that the element of fear has crept in again.

For instance, a potential career changer may initially fear the unknown in general and may have feelings of inadequacy. Once that individual has gotten unstuck from his old situation and has taken the direction necessary to actually start the career change process, more fears could arise at different points along the way. At the learning or retraining stage for the new career, he may fear that he will fail to learn the new trade, that he won't pass the retraining courses, or that he'll lack sufficient financial resources to see the training period through.

Once the learning path is over that same individual may experience fears about a lack of good job opportunities, his competency on the job once hired, potential rejection by new associates, or the level of his income, especially at the beginning stages.

As you can see, the career changer is faced with different kinds of fears throughout the whole process of the transition. At each stage, people in transition must learn to face any attendant fears that come with the stage they are at in their bid to enter a new smooth, paved road.

As discussed in Chapter 5, you can face your fears (at whatever stage) by first identifying them and calling them by name, questioning the assumptions on which the fears are based, presenting yourself with contrary views that transcend those assumptions, and continuing to affirm the positive views.

Getting to the New Place during Multiple Transitions

In the introduction you met Samantha, who experienced multiple transitions, one after the other—the loss of her mother and her fiancé, the loss of her material possessions to fire, and a delay in her career advancement—all within a short period of time. Just as Samantha was taking some initial steps forward from the first transition, she got stuck again in another muddy path.

Just like Samantha, you may have become unstuck from one muddy path only to experience another transition before you could master a new smooth, paved road. Multiple entries onto and exits out of the muddy path may leave you feeling exhausted. However, rest assured that there is hope. You can acquire the sanity and strength to untie the knots of even the concurrent transitions. Your wisdom to get unstuck lies in the fact that you can isolate the issues surrounding these transitions and sort them into a prioritized list. Recognize that you do not have to deal with all of the issues at once.

As you view your prioritized list and plan your actions on a step-by-step basis, you will begin to move forward. As you define your momentum in such a way that you do not become overwhelmed, the inertia created by the complexity of your situation will be eliminated. As you enjoy forward progress in small steps, stay motivated. Ultimately, you will begin to acquire more power to move even further ahead.

In this chapter I have discussed how to take action on the option you have chosen as a way to resume your journey. I highlighted the issues associated with designing the action steps, and I elaborated on the processes of finding a new identity and the strength you need to move toward your new goal.

Now that you have started moving, how do you build upon the foundation you have laid to ensure further success? This question will be addressed in the next chapter.

Wisdom Tips

Use laughter to lessen the stress of your situation or problem. When you laugh at yourself and your problems, you are able to deal with that pain in a focused but lighter fashion, putting you in a better position to move through the situation causing the pain.

Use the support of discerning companions. The moral support of a listening ear offered by a discerning companion-friend, family or community member - can be of great help in maintaining your sanity and strength as you move on.

Power Tips

Forgive and release the past. Stop giving your power away to bitterness, anger, and many other negative emotions.

Maintain your physical and mental well-being. Keeping physically fit and nourishing your body and spirit will help give you the reserves of energy you need for moving on.

Chapter 8

HOW DO I STABILIZE MYSELF IN MY NEW POSITION?

Having set new goals for your new journey and having acquired the power to take the action steps required to meet these goals, you are now poised for continuous motion in the new direction you have chosen. However, continuity does not just happen. To experience steady motion on your new journey, you will need to put in more effort on top of the initial effort it took to get you going. Having some stability in your new position requires more action on your part. The issue of maintaining continuous motion is the subject of this chapter.

Consider What Stability Means to You

The word "stabilize" is defined as "to make steady; to make unwavering, constant, and firm." This position sounds reassuring; we human beings desire stability in some form or another. This is especially true if you have been through a rough time or a challenging life or career transition. When you are stabilized, there is less stress. In addition, "stability" could indicate when opposing forces are balanced in a particular situation; that is, when no extrinsic factors, such as influences from outsiders or your environment, are pulling away from intrinsic factors, such as your inner struggles or your personal likes and dislikes.

Considering this, after all you have been through to resume your life's journey, the tendency is that you will want to stabilize yourself in your new position—and this desire is a very good one. However, your perspective on stability is very important and it may differ from one life transition to the next. It is, therefore, imperative in your move toward stability that you take time to ask the question:

- What does stability mean to me in this current scenario?

When you answer this thought-provoking question you are more poised to establish yourself in your new position. When you define what stability means to you in your forward move, you will be able to run at your pace and gather the momentum required to move forward successfully without getting overwhelmed again.

Diane's Perspective of Stability

Diane has taken a number of forward steps since coming to terms with her current situation. She has done a lot of research into the resources available for managing her condition of lupus. Her sister also comes to live with her for a few months after her diagnosis. This helps a lot in the initial phases of the change. Diane also enlists the services of a nurse to help her with many issues of mobility.

After the initial upheaval, Diane considers what to do with her business venture. She had always had great fulfillment with the venture. To close it down altogether would be devastating. That would be another huge loss and Diane is not sure she can handle that at this phase of her transition. There would be too many factors to adjust to all at once. At the same time, Diane knows it will be quite challenging to continue to run the business in the same way she had. She needs to modify her approach, since she does not have the vigor she had before the diagnosis. Diane feels that once her health stabilizes she will be able to work on a new approach for her business.

So Diane works on goals related to making her present health condition more stable. She takes her prescribed medications and keeps her doctor appointments. She does exercises to ease her joint pains, takes time to rest between major activities, and continues to affirm to herself that she is going to make it. Though it may take some effort and might require a new route, Diane feels confident that she is going to get back to her business and be fulfilled at it again in the near future.

Out of Alignment!

On resuming his journey and traveling for a few miles in his chosen direction, Brian the truck driver suddenly feels there is something weird about the motion of his truck. The truck seems a little unbalanced and its movement is wobbly. Brian pulls over to the side of the road to check what is happening. To his surprise, he finds that his wheels are out of alignment.

"Oh!" Brian says to himself, "The impact of the truck hitting the potholes must have caused the wheels to go out of alignment." Brian decides that the best approach is to find a nearby garage to correct the situation. Fortunately, he had just seen a road sign indicating there is a gas station nearby. He drives slowly to the station and asks to have all of his wheels properly aligned.

Bring Your Core Values into Focus

In Chapter 6 you had a chance to work on discovering your life's purpose in your new circumstances. I mentioned that this is an essential step whether you were doing it for the first time or reevaluating a purpose you'd identified in the past.

Based on your newly defined life's purpose, you have drawn out a new set of goals and action plans to achieve the dreams you have for a new, smooth paved road (Chapter 7). You have even begun to achieve some of these goals as you worked on discovering a new identity for moving on.

However, some things may still not be working out properly. Just like Brian discovered his truck had a wobbly motion, you may experience a reduction in speed on your new smooth, paved road. Some unidentified factors seem to be creeping up and causing you to slow down again.

There could be a number of reasons for this decrease in your momentum. One could be that your new goals or the means you have identified for achieving them are not in alignment with your core values. Just as the unsteady motion of Brian's truck was caused by non-aligned wheels, your slow progress may be due to non-alignment of your goals and action steps with your core values. So what are your values?

Clarifying your core values

Your core values depict who you are as a person, what you value about life, and the way you like things to operate. They are important components of who you are, and any clashes or non-alignment with your core values may make you feel unsteady and lack inner harmony.

Values are such things as integrity, honesty, productivity, adventure, risk taking, being organized, freedom, connection, and innovation. Knowing your values will help you to further embrace the big picture of your life's purpose. It will also be of great assistance in determining your action steps and the methods to use to execute them.

Here is a basic way to clarify your values. Step back into your past and identify a peak moment in your life when you felt quite fulfilled and everything was rewarding.

- What was happening at that moment?
- Which values were being honored at that moment?

Another approach is to step into the past and identify a low moment in your life when you felt totally frustrated and unhappy. Now the question to ask is:

- Which values were not being honored at that moment?

Those values that you feel were being suppressed must be important to you.

As values are central to the core of your being, it is essential that you take time to align the approach you use to achieve your new goals with these values. This should eliminate any further decrease in your momentum.

On Being Both the Leader and the Driver

You may be trying to get back into some social circles after losing a valuable romantic relationship. Perhaps your goals include meeting new people and ultimately going on some new dates. These are good goals to set in your particular situation. However, if in trying to meet new people you have been taking all leads that come your way without any screening, you might be setting yourself up for an incident that induces new lethargy.

You will need to view how you meet new people and who you are arranging to meet through the lens of your core values, which could be such things as integrity, freedom, and adventure. You are the leader in your new situation, the leader of this process of moving on. So, take the lead by aligning your goals and methods of achieving them with your core values.

Another reason you might be experiencing lethargy could be that you are not taking the proper position in the driver's seat of your new life's purpose. This might be especially true if the stimulus for your life transition has its roots in the fact that some third party drew your previous life plan. This third party may be someone of great influence in your life such as a parent, spouse, or community leader who tried to impose their wishes or plan upon you.

As you work on the action steps you have mapped out on your new route, it is wise to repeat that situation. Thus, for the new set of goals you have proposed to achieve, take your full position in the driver's seat; sit upright and get your whole body and mind ready for the full range of actions required for driving.

When you are both the leader and driver on your new journey, you are able to incorporate your core values into it. You are able to take full ownership and have more focus on achieving your goals. And with this kind of posture, you are more likely to enjoy the journey and, therefore, eliminate new blockades.

Reinforce What You Have Already Established

Having aligned your goal-achievement process with your values, and having taken the leader and driver position, you are ready to strengthen what you have established and thereby further stabilize your new position. As you continue to take more of the steps that yield good results, you reinforce those results.

Continue to work on areas of your life that were previously made stagnant as a result of the transition. Continue what you started when you reactivated and plugged back the power into such areas as relationships, family and family responsibilities, intellectual pursuits, spirituality, work, colleagues, and physical fitness and health.

You will also be buttressing what you have started by continuing to take charge in your new situation. Continue to say no to what you need to say no to. If you have set goals about reducing your expenses to match your means in your new situation, you will need to continue to say no to all indulgences or expenses that do not support this new goal.

Continue to say yes to what you need to say yes to. If you are on your way toward finding a new job after a job loss, you need to continue to say yes to networking and positive interactions with other people.

One essential way of reinforcing what you have already established is to work on developing your new identity.

Develop Your Newly Discovered Identity

In Chapter 7 I discussed different ways of finding a new identity. To strengthen the new identity you have discovered you need to first embrace it and then develop it further. New lifestyle patterns are not always appealing, and some take time to form. In embracing your new identity you need to continue to welcome your new patterns of behavior. You can even make it more tangible by writing an affirmation statement for your new lifestyle pattern and sharing it with family and friends.

Developing your identity further also means you are growing in it, getting more comfortable in it, and maturing it. Be intentional about creating time for your newly discovered opportunities. Make time for activities that boost your self-esteem. Spend time developing those new friendships. Give your attention to community involvements that support you in your altered role or status. For instance, if you have become a single parent after losing a partner, pay attention to those meetings that support you in your altered parenting role. Continue to tap into avenues for spiritual renewal.

As you take steps to develop your new identity, it will become more real to you. It will become more natural to see yourself in it. And as you further develop it, this new identity becomes you—the authentic new you.

Reevaluate Periodically to Assess Your Progress

In Chapter 7 I discussed the importance of setting SMART goals for initiating your new journey. This tool helped bring to reality your aspirations for a new smooth, paved road. SMART goals equip you for success because, among other things, they help you set an expected time for completing the action steps to achieve a particular goal.

You may have been able to achieve some level of success since you began to set those goals. But there are more goals to set and action steps to design to reach your new destination via that new smooth, paved road. How do you ensure you are on track in your journey? How do you measure success along the way?

The best way to measure success is through periodic evaluations of your goals. These evaluations are meant to help you determine your progress on the action steps you designed. These evaluations are best done at intervals of time set by you. In setting the intervals, be sure to allow adequate time to perform enough action steps so that you'll have something meaningful to evaluate.

During your periodic evaluations, spend time analyzing the action steps for your goals. Take a look at the ones you have completed. Congratulate yourself for this and celebrate your small wins. Then take time to analyze the ones that were due but have not yet been completed. Ask probing questions about the possible reasons for their incompletion. Then take a big-picture view of your whole set of future goals and look at them through the lens of your recently completed goals. Ask yourself whether there are actions you should continue doing in the same way, actions you should be doing more of, or actions you should stop doing altogether. Also ask yourself whether you need to change the approach you are using to ensure better results for the new action steps.

These periodic evaluations will help you monitor your success on a goal-by-goal basis. Apart from these individual assessments, you may include some time for big-picture analysis during your periodic evaluation period. For this general overview of your progress, find a quiet spot for reflection and ask:

- What am I becoming?
- What am I building?

It's fine to separate this big-picture overview analysis from your goal-by-goal analysis. The most important thing is that you schedule time for it.

Deal With New Obstacles That Come up on Your New Journey

Since you are on a new journey, you are prone to encountering new obstacles in your way. The fact that you have resumed your journey on another path makes you vulnerable to new barriers. In fact, you may experience another change or transition. The only constant in life is change, and even a steady journey encounters new change from time to time. You will have to navigate your way around these new changes or obstacles in a manner similar to the one you used to get unstuck from the previous one. Apply the principles highlighted in the previous chapters to overcome any new barriers.

Elena Sets Her Pace to Fit Her Definition of Stability

Elena knows things are much different for her now. It has been eighteen months since Hurricane Katrina and she has come a long way since then. Although there's no way the huge jolt she suffered can be erased, she has managed to make some progress. Now living in Chicago, where she and other survivors of the hurricane were rehabilitated, she has started making new friends in her neighborhood. She has a new home, which was initially rented to her for free after her arrival in the city. She also has a new church and a new job at a hotel restaurant.

She had landed the job after taking some evening classes to brush up on her skills for the hospitality industry. In Elena's timeline, this job will be a temporary one. She still has an unquenched dream to start a new diner in a suitable location. But that is in the future. At the present moment, Elena's focus is on building new social relationships in her new environment. She has gradually defined what stability means to her at this phase of her transition. She has also learned that, although the transition is taking some time, it is better to take it at her own pace to ensure stability in the new future she is building.

Cast a New Vision of the Future

You have moved from having a new sense of direction and a new route map (Chapter 6) to having a new set of goals and power to move. You have gathered some momentum (Chapter 7) and have started stabilizing yourself on your new route. Now the question comes to mind:

- How long will it take to get to my new destination?

This question calls for a fresh vision of your journey and destination.

Before heading out on your original journey you had a vision of where you expected to be in a certain period of time. Now, with all the modifications, you need to cast a new vision of where (i.e., which point on your new mapped-out route) you expect to be in your new journey after a given period of time. This envisioning process—I call it vision casting—will help you achieve great success on the new smooth, paved road you are now on.

To cast a vision of your new journey, ask yourself the question:

- If I have all the resources (financial, intellectual, etc.) that I need for this new journey and I have all the time to focus on it, where do I expect to be three years from now?

Now step into the future and envision a day five years from now. Imagine you are looking back from that date to now, and ask:

- What needs to have happened over the last five years for me to feel happy with my progress?

As you answer these questions you will be able to cast a new vision for your journey. Write the answers down and use them to draw a set of vision statements for various areas of your life; you can merge these statements into an overall life vision.

Regularly review this new vision statement, especially during your periodic evaluations. This will help you keep track of your success on your new paved road.

The process of developing a fresh vision of your destination will empower you to continue working on the steps toward it. This in turn will position you for making it through to a new you.

Make it through to a New You

The preceding sections explored the issue of stabilizing yourself in your new journey through further development of what you established after getting unstuck and through periodic evaluations of your progress. But how do you ensure you make it through to your new destination via the new smooth, paved road?

You can ensure your success in a number of ways:

- Maintaining continuous motion in the same direction

- Empowering yourself for more success through celebrations of your progress

- Taking ownership of your new identity

Our human tendency to resist change and the unfamiliar remains a solid factor even during the middle phases of change. Despite the fact that you have already achieved some goals in your new journey and you are beginning to have some success, you may still be tempted slip back into the old way of doing things. You do not want a situation where you move forward by three steps but then slip back by two steps. Such a pattern of motion will not augur success in your new journey.

I must reiterate that at times it is necessary to go back and view previous lines of questioning to help you discover better lines of action. However, when you do go back to review what you have done during this transition journey, it is essential not to stay stuck in the position you previously navigated your way out of. It is essential to shift gears back to where you were and always maintain motion in the forward direction. Avoid getting stuck again in old familiar ways.

Here are some tips that will help you maintain your movement forward.

Nullify ghosts of your past

Ghosts of your past life may appear on your new route, especially in the middle phase of change. These may be influences from contacts or physical items from the past that tend to haunt you and make you question your sanity regarding the new approach, direction, and journey you are now taking, despite the fact that you have had some great successes on this new path.

These thoughts may harass or beguile you about the new direction you are taking. They may try to persuade you that you are nuts and are missing out by forsaking all your old ways. At times they may even try to encourage you to go back to things you have successfully said bye–bye to. They may attempt to convince you that it's going to cost you more money and/or time to achieve good results or break even on your new pathway compared to returning to your old path.

Maybe you have decided to change your career in order to spend more time with your family. This change requires retraining on your part and you have settled on taking an online course for the next two years. However, midway to achieving this goal, some ghosts from your past show up and try to convince you that you are losing your seniority status in your old profession. "Would it not be easier for you to stop pursuing this strange new career and pick up a job that is easily available in your previous career?" they ask you.

Ghosts of the past can be even more terrifying in cases of imposed life transitions, such as a divorce. The fear they cause is often gripping because you know there is actually no way to revive the past.

So what are you to do when such ghosts come your way when you are concentrating hard on establishing yourself on a new path? How do you neutralize their effect and thereby maintain your sanity? How do you get rid of them and enjoy steady forward motion?

You need to firmly invalidate the effects of the ghosts and abolish their influence. You can do this by:

- Enhancing the actions you are taking on your new path

- Continuing to affirm your new intentions to keep walking in the new direction

- Continuing to remove any items from your old route that are still lingering around you

- Increasing your efforts to envision your desired future

- Furnishing and equipping your physical environment so it will continue to nourish you as you attempt to attain your goals

- Moving away from the old environment if necessary

Empower yourself for more success by celebrating small wins along the way

As I mentioned above in the section on periodic evaluations, take time to celebrate your progress as you move toward your new way of life. You may not have reached your overall goal yet, but you are not the same as you were during the first moments of your transition.

For instance, if you lost a business relationship, you may have just been able to restructure your organizational infrastructure. You may have been able to modify your employees' job functions or outsource some of the functions performed by the partner you lost. That is worth celebrating. Celebrating the small achievements you make on your journey will help reaffirm your confidence that you will be successful in your transition. It will help you gather momentum for more achievements.

Take ownership of your new identity

You have embraced your new identity through various means. You have spent considerable time developing this new identity. So continue to take ownership of it. Move on with this identity. Continue to affirm that this is the new you. Let the world know that this new you is authentic and real. Doing this will position you to keep moving forward, and that is the position you need to maintain—forward motion. In addition, keep striving to learn and experience new things that are in line with your desired goals.

As you stabilize yourself in your new position you will become more established on the new route you have taken. You will be more confident of your new identity. You will be positioned for more success and able to stay on top of new challenges that come your way.

While going through this transition you have not lived in a vacuum. You have been influenced by people in your circles of influence—your family, close friends, neighborhood, and community at large. Some of these people might have helped you through moments of despair and struggle. Some may have even mentored you on your way back to the new smooth, paved road you are now on. How do you give back to these people? How do you impact your circles of influence with the lessons you have learned during your transition? The next chapter provides some perspectives on this line of questioning.

Wisdom Tips

Periodic re-evaluation to assess your progress is a useful tool for stabilizing yourself in your new position.

Cast a new vision of your future from your new vantage position. This will further help in stabilizing you on your new smooth paved road.

Power Tips

Define what stability means to you in your forward move. This will help you run at your pace and gather the momentum required to move forward successfully without getting overwhelmed again.

Celebrate small wins along the way. This will provide you with motivation to continue on your new smooth paved road.

Chapter 9

HOW DO I IMPACT MY COMMUNITY WITH THE LESSONS LEARNED THROUGH MY EXPERIENCE?

In the last set of chapters you have gone through a process of liberating yourself from the sticky factors associated with a life- or career-changing event. You have been able to identify a new direction in which to continue your journey. You have even gone on to set new goals and achieve some successes in this new direction. Now that you are gradually stabilizing yourself in your new position, what else can you do to solidify your stance? How can you make more meaning from your experiences? How can you add more value to what you have already begun? And how can you be more fulfilled in your new stabilized position? The current chapter explores these issues in depth.

Paul Decides to Volunteer
His Time at a Special Sporting Event

Paul, the former car salesman from previous chapters, is able to get a temporary job through his networking efforts. He still has it in mind to pick up a professional course in business and computing, but the temporary job offer as a front-line salesperson for a dairy company will provide him and his family with some regular income for the time being.

He and Kate readjust their family budget and recalculate their finances to adapt to their changed circumstances. One of the changes involves Kate's hip surgery; she has to go through rehabilitation and this involves a number of sessions with a physical therapist.

It is during one of these sessions that Paul learns that the center needs people to help out with a sports event for the physically challenged. Although his life is not the way it used to be, Paul has an innate urge to volunteer his time at this event. Yes, a number of things in his life are not completely stabilized, but he has learned that helping others can also make one's own life better. So, he pitches in at this event for the physically challenged.

While volunteering, Paul recollects that an instructor in the job search class he had attended had said that volunteering could expand his network and help him meet new people who may be able to assist in his job search. Paul had also taken to heart the attendant warning that he should watch his motives for volunteering. He remembers that he should not make it all about the job search, but to open himself to meaningful relationships.

These tips from the job search instructor are relevant, but Paul knows that the sheer joy he will get from helping others will be worth the effort. He also thinks that this volunteer activity will help him relate to Kate during her continued rehabilitation from the surgery. He is certain that working with people who have physical challenges will equip him to support Kate at this phase of her own transition.

Sharing Blesses Others as Well as Yourself

Paul has to move out of his comfort zone to give of himself at the sports event for the physically challenged. In similar ways, you may be moving out of your comfort zone to share with others. However, you will find that sharing has lots of benefits, not only for the people or cause you are giving your time to, but also for you, the giver. Sharing will open new avenues for becoming even more stabilized in your new circumstances.

As you interact with others in this way, the new social interactions will boost your self-esteem. This aspect is even more relevant if your transition is a relationship-based one, such as the loss of a spouse or dear friend. In addition, the sense of accomplishment and the joy of seeing the impact you have on others will lift your inner self and reignite your passion for life. You will experience more vitality when you see the positive results of your input in the lives of others. All of these positive effects will empower you to pursue the goals you have set for yourself in other areas.

Shift Your Mindset toward a Dream That Is Bigger than You

You might agree with the benefits of sharing, but perhaps you are still brooding over the whole idea of sharing at this stage of your life. You might be saying to yourself, "I am barely recovered from the effects of the transition. How am I supposed to give of myself to others?"

This kind of mental struggle can be due to a number of reasons. One may be that you are still harboring resentment toward someone or something that might have been responsible for the transition you experienced.

Maybe you have forgiven the past, as I discussed in Chapter 7, but you have not fully released the stimulus responsible for your change. In this case, it will be extremely difficult for you to embrace the idea of caring for something or someone else even though you have moved on in many other aspects of your life. But sharing with individuals who have no responsibility for your changed circumstances is a good way to ensure total release. At a later stage you might become more confident of sharing even with the cause of your transition.

Another reason why the concept of sharing may not sound reasonable to you at this phase is that society puts a "fragile, handle with care" label on people going through tough transitions. Although people's raw emotions manifest more during tough times, this does not preclude you from taking some steps in the direction of sharing. Depending on your situation, this type of activity or goal could even be vital to your healing process.

Related to this societal perception of your vulnerability is our innate human tendency. Your mental mode may not be geared to thinking beyond yourself since you have just emerged or are still trying hard to emerge from a not-so-easy transition experience. You may want to keep to yourself and reserve your energy for things that are directly for you. However, this mindset is self-limiting, and you do not have to stay stuck in its restrictions. You can be bold and take on a new mindset that is more liberating. You can decide to think outside yourself and see a more global picture.

This outward-facing mindset provides a framework that is larger than you because it pulls you toward goals you would not normally set out to achieve. It provides more opportunities for you to stretch yourself, thereby putting you in a stance for more achievements. In turn, these achievements will open new doors of opportunity in realms that you would not otherwise have thought possible. Such new opportunities may occur in areas of your life beyond just those touched by your life transition, providing avenues for balanced growth and making you a better person as a whole.

As you embrace the concept of sharing, you will see clearly which avenues are open for you to give of yourself even at this stage of your new journey.

Discover the Many Options for Sharing or Giving

Sharing or giving of yourself can take forms as varied as volunteering your time on a one-on-one basis to regular participation in community projects. Simple sharing of your time with family members that goes outside the realm of what you normally did before the transition will also expand your reach. Offering to babysit, attend a PTA meeting, or go to a piano recital on behalf of someone who can't make it may be as important as getting involved in huge community projects. The important factor is the ability to give.

Getting involved with your community can also take various shapes. You may decide to volunteer for those in need of general amenities of life, or those who are experiencing challenges in other ways than you have experienced. It could be as simple as helping out in a soup kitchen for the homeless or leading a group of youngsters on a camping trip. It could mean offering your expertise to a non-profit organization that needs such assistance but cannot afford to hire you. Or it could mean signing up for a shopping assistance service for seniors. Extending yourself to help others in these avenues is a means of personal growth for you in general. The maturity that comes from looking outside yourself and focusing your attention on the needs of others can serve as a buoy to keep you afloat on a general basis.

On the other hand, you may also give of yourself in specific ways that are directly related to the experience you have just navigated through. You can serve as a group leader in a community organization that supports people going through divorce or other relationship breakdown. You may serve in job clubs for those who have just lost their jobs. If your kids are grown or you are free from core family responsibilities, you may even volunteer to work outside your community in areas that serve people you are interested in sharing your story or expertise with. The survivor of a hurricane may be interested in traveling with a disaster relief organization like the Red Cross to help more recent survivors of another natural disaster.

If you are a vocal person, you may be interested in advocating for vulnerable people in your community in general or for those passing through a life transition that you have just been through. For instance, someone who lost her husband to an unfortunate accident instigated by a group of rebellious teenagers opted to spend her time speaking about and advocating for restorative justice, a means whereby the perpetrators of such offenses could be reabsorbed into society and lead meaningful lives. Not only did this course of action help a number of teenagers become more responsible members of society, but the woman advocate also found more meaning and fulfillment in her new circumstances.

The opportunities are endless to share and give of yourself. What is important is that you are willing to explore such avenues of giving back.

Getting Involved Helps Harry Reignite His Passion for Life

Harry, who lost his wife of forty years, has over the course of time acknowledged that moving on from the loss does not necessarily mean he is dishonoring his wife. In fact, to the contrary; many of the processes he has been through to discover and embrace a new identity have in one way or the other served as means of honoring Debra. One powerful sentence that has been a source of empowerment for Harry is, "If Debra were here, she would love that I am happy and living a life of fulfillment." Saying this to himself has offered a great perspective to Harry on numerous occasions.

With this kind of positive attitude Harry has been able to achieve some successes on the new journey he is now taking. He has signed on as an instructor for the e-learning course he had been contemplating just before Debra passed away. He has designed new courses for an interactive online environment, finding his background knowledge to be helpful even though this is different from any instruction he has done before. He has also become more active in his church. All of these things have helped stabilize Harry's journey in his new circumstances.

However, when looking objectively at what has contributed immensely to his sense of fulfillment, Harry realizes that one project stands out from the rest: his involvement with the Hospital Foundation. Since Debra's passing, Harry has always been curious about what had caused her sudden death after an infection that had seemed so trivial. He had been told that Debra's death was due to a secondary infection superimposed on the first one, so over time he has talked to many medical doctors and medical researchers both at the local hospital and globally through the Internet.

It was during one of these talks that he learned of the Hospital Foundation's efforts to raise funds for research into the cause of the secondary infection. Harry decided to volunteer some of his time with this foundation. Initially he helped with some of the research, but eventually opportunities opened up to become even more involved. He is now fully involved with fundraising and other management functions at the Hospital Foundation, and is a significant voice for them in his community and elsewhere.

The more he gives of himself in this regard, the more Harry experiences healing. His giving back to his community has indeed helped reignite Harry's zest for life and increase his enjoyment of life in his new circumstances.

Plug into the Amazing, Life-transforming Power of Stories

As mentioned above, one of the ways you can give back to your community is by sharing your story—the story of your struggles and how you have emerged (or are still emerging) from the challenges you have experienced. No matter which avenue you use to share your story, there is tremendous power in this activity.

When you share your story in a group setting, it helps people connect with one another and with you. If your audience can relate to your story it helps them recognize that they are not alone in their struggles. This kind of awareness gives people hope and an assurance that there is a way out of their situation. It encourages them to take action, action that also positions them for success. This in turn multiplies your success.

"No man is an island" is a well-known cliché. But how true it is! The fact that you have been able to overcome the challenge of your transition and are now enjoying success on a new smooth, paved road is great. What is even greater is that there are people who can benefit from your experience if you share it with them. So aim to live not for yourself only but for others as well. Go on and tell your story to people in forums or support groups who are facing similar situations.

Apart from avenues that involve your physical presence, our high-tech world provides numerous other opportunities for you to share your story. You can write a blog, participate in Internet forums, post to websites. You can also share through audio and video if you are so inclined.

No matter where or how you share your story, recognize that people will connect with you and you will have an even greater impact if you are authentic. Be genuine when sharing your story. People will see through you if you are not. Share your struggles as well as the successes you have achieved in the process of navigating your way through change. This will make your story more relevant and easier to grasp than a polished tale that mentions only your successes.

Savannah Realizes a Great Sense of Liberation as She Shares Her Story

Savannah, who has been navigating her way through the challenges of divorce, is approached by Cindy, a representative from a women's health organization who is planning a conference on women, family life, and careers. The organization is looking for professionals who are experts on the topic, as well as working-class women whose careers have been impacted by changes in their family life.

Cindy had gotten Savannah's contact information from a former work colleague who had raved about how magnificently Savannah had come out of her divorce. Savannah remembers that this work contact had told her about this conference a number of times in the past, but now the real invitation has come. Knowing that this is Savannah's private life, Cindy quickly adds that Savannah should not feel pressured or sorry if she is not ready to go public with her experience. "However, there are many women out there who could benefit from your story," Cindy says, "and this forum is a good one in which to share it."

At first it is difficult for Savannah to visualize the scenario of a talk on her life. How can she stand in front of an audience of over five hundred people and tell them about the unpleasant things that happened in her own family? After a few days of struggling with the idea, Savannah finally resolves to give the talk. It is not easy at first, but as she settles into the talk Savannah feels more comfortable with the women. She narrates her struggles, especially with her identity, the issues about single parenting and sharing joint custody with Fred, and the changes she has had to make in her work schedule.

The good and surprising thing is that she is able to share her intimate feelings with this group of strangers. What's more, after she finishes the talk Savannah feels a heave of relief and freedom all about her. This relief is much greater than anything she had ever experienced giving presentations during her career as a senior medical representative. The current relief is not associated with the relief she got after a public speech; in fact she was used to public speeches in her career. This freedom is something different that she cannot explain.

She would never have guessed that the mere fact that she was willing to make herself vulnerable and share her story could bring such a sense of freedom to her. Yes, she has come a long way since she received those divorce papers. She has waded through the muddy waters and found some new direction for her life. She has achieved other new successes in her resumed journey, but what she experiences after the talk at the conference is unparalleled. It is as if she has doubled her vitality for life.

Ryan Becomes More Stable by Giving Back

Ryan, the computer associate who lost the use of his leg in a workplace accident, goes forward with his career change plan. He takes some community courses in entrepreneurship and uses the resources of his city's chamber of commerce to find more information on the whole process. He explores options as to which kind of services he can offer. There are many avenues in his field, but Ryan knows that, in his new state, he has to define what is practical and what is not.

So Ryan settles for social media and search engine optimization consulting. He updates himself on which aspects to target and what kind of industries to offer services for. Since this is an actively growing field there is an enormous amount of information to research, but the urge for independence keeps Ryan going. In addition, he gets some help from people in his industry. Networking with contacts he had made in his former job and with colleagues from his college days also proves helpful.

Ryan gradually sets up his start-up company and takes on this new direction with wholehearted vigor. While the process is demanding in some ways, Ryan also finds a much-needed renewed zest for life in a side project. During the course of his research Ryan had come across two associations offering services for people who are physically challenged. He signed on as a member of these two associations and has since been able to interact with the administrators and leaders.

When he finds out that one of these associations needs help managing and updating its website, Ryan is gladly willing to help. He takes on this responsibility and finds much fulfillment in a boost to his self-esteem. By giving back to an organization that serves him and the people he has now come to appreciate more, Ryan is able to acquire more strength for his new direction in life.

This chapter has explained the importance of moving out of your comfort zone to share with members of your community even as you emerge from the muddy paths of life transition. The process of giving back helps boost your self-esteem and provides a new means of fulfillment for you. This, in turns, increases your stability on your new smooth, paved road. In addition, you are impacting the lives of many more people for good with your positive influence.

On another note, sharing and getting involved helps you become fully alive. Your passion for life is reignited as you help others through various means. Taking on dreams that are larger than you expands your reach. This puts you in a position where you can continue to multiply your wisdom and strength, a process that should keep you on top in the many new journeys you may take.

Wisdom Tips

Take on a liberating mindset of thinking outside of yourself and your needs. Shift your mindset towards sharing with others and giving back. Such an outward-facing mindset will stretch you and thereby put you in a stance for more achievements and personal growth.

The process of giving back helps boost your self-esteem and provides a new means of fulfillment for you. In addition, you are impacting the lives of many more people for good with your positive influence.

Power Tips

Sharing blesses others as well as yourself. Move out of your comfort zone and share with others even during this stage of your experience.

Sharing will open new avenues for becoming even more stabilized in your new circumstances.

Tell your stories to others. Share about your transition, your struggles and victories. Experience the transforming power of your sharing in the lives of your audience.

Chapter 10

CONCLUSION

You have come a long way through this book. At the beginning I explained how easy it is to carry on daily living when there is some form of constancy in your life. I described this phase of life where you are comfortable and able to plan for the next day with ease as journeying on a smooth, paved road. I emphasized how this state is somewhat elusive because life is full of changes. In fact, change is a necessary part of life. Change gives birth to life and life gives birth to change.

So it is imperative to know how to handle periods of change in your life. I explained the concept of change readiness, an attitude that will make you more adaptable to regular change events in your life. Preparing for the inevitability of change includes deliberately including simple detours from your routine, thereby creating intentional change and making you more comfortable with it.

I also reiterated that no matter how change ready you are, you are still susceptible to huge changes that are earth-shattering and that can impact the course of your life. Such huge changes include marriage (or remarriage), divorce, becoming a parent, job loss, career moves, death of a loved one, retirement, and cross-county or international relocations.

This book has focused on how to navigate through these life-changing events and come out on top on the other side. The process of navigating through the muddy path of transition is an evolving progression of search and discovery on your part. This seeking-and-finding process is built on a framework of seven powerful questions that create the awareness you need to get unstuck from the muddy path and that inspire you to take the necessary actions to move forward with your life on a new smooth, paved road.

Seven Powerful Questions for Navigating through Change

At the onset of a life transition or career change you are often bombarded with an overwhelming feeling of helplessness, which often presents itself as inertia. At this stage you tend to be stuck, because there are many sticky factors immobilizing you and pinning you in the same position—as exemplified by the truck stuck on a muddy path. During this stuck phase, the essential tools you need are those that will help you get the confusion out so you gain a better understanding of your situation. Therefore, you ask the questions:

- Where am I?

- How did I get here?

- Who am I in this present situation?

Powerful Question One
Where am I?

This question is aimed at eliminating the confusion that arises just after a life-changing event diverts you from your smooth, paved road onto a muddy path. Not having anticipated the event, you are jolted and thrown into a state of confusion and shock. For anything meaningful to happen after this you need to emerge from a confused state and become alert enough to gain an understanding of your new surroundings and bearings. This is an essential step, because this recognition will serve as a fulcrum from which you can launch any future action.

Powerful Question Two
How did I get here?

When you become aware of your location and bearings as they relate to the muddy path you have entered, you need to figure out how you got to that place. This process of retracing your journey will help you establish the causes of your transition. Having this information will enable you to identify the sticky factors that might be keeping you in the stuck position and what you can do to get rid of them. The knowledge of who or what caused your transition is also vital for the healing you might need to move through the transition process.

Powerful Question Three
Who am I in this present situation?

The fact that some things about your situation have changed means there is a form of discontinuity in your person, either physically or in other areas. This discontinuity causes a crisis in your awareness of who you really are, thus impacting your identity. This change in your identity creates further confusion, and you need to recognize the fact that the old you is gone. You need to become aware of how the transition has affected different parts of your identity—physical self/ self-esteem, intellectual, family, spiritual, economic, and social. This inquiry helps you identify what has changed and ultimately come to terms with the fact that you can no longer use the old identity in your forward move.

The three questions you ask while at the stuck phase create awareness and provoke thoughts that initiate clarity on your condition. They help you establish your location and bearings and come to terms with the fact that your identity has changed. In other words, these questions instigate your search for a means of getting unstuck.

As a result, you become ready to take on the simple but powerful question:

- How do I get unstuck?

Powerful Question Four
How do I get unstuck?

This question is at the very heart of the transition process. The fact is, if you don't get unstuck you will remain in the same position. You need to find out what to do to get rid of the inertia that the change has created and thereby initiate some movement.

The previous three questions should have prepared you to tackle this essential inquiry. Using the facts you have gathered from your answers you are able to decipher what you need to stop doing and what you need to start doing in order to get rid of the sticky factors holding you down in that muddy path. The list of things to take on might include creating the right environment and shifting your mindset to accommodate new perspectives. Powerful Question 4 may also stimulate you to seek the outside help you might need to get unstuck, such as help from the community or professional coaches.

Unstuck! That is powerful and exciting. But what do you do with your new situation? The obvious answer is that you move on from the muddy path. The powerful questions for the moving-on phase are:

- Where do I go now?

- How do I get to that new place?

- How do I stabilize myself in my new position?

Powerful Question Five
Where do I go now?

You need to know where to go to be able to plan your forward journey. This question helps you analyze whether you can afford to keep going in the same direction and/or destination or whether you need to go to a different place. Your decision will be based on your answers to the previous questions about what has changed in your situation and which parts of your identity have been affected by the change.

An essential part of this inquiry is taking time to envision a new place that you can go given your new set of circumstances. Once you are able to narrow down your options on such a destination, you are now ready to take on the next line of probing: the means of getting to that new place.

Powerful Question Six
How do I get to that new place?

This inquiry is a necessary follow-up on the previous one. Having envisioned a new place, it becomes obvious there is a gap between where you are and that new place. To bridge that gap you will need to carry out some action steps that will move you toward the new destination and ultimately get you to that place. You need to map a new route for your journey or modify the previous one. The question will stimulate you to research new options, analyze them, and decide on which one to pursue. It will instigate you to set new goals related to your new route and delineate ways of achieving those goals so that your forward move will become a reality.

The question also stimulates you to seek means of getting the needed energy boost required for this phase. You may discover a new identity as you revive those things that were left stagnant as a result of the transition. In addition, the probing will help you delineate which momentum-creating tools you may need to move forward.

Once you get moving you will begin to achieve some successes on the new smooth, paved road you have entered.

Powerful Question Seven
How do I stabilize myself in my new position?

The beginning of a new journey is important and indicates progress on your path. However, it is not the end. For your new destination to become a reality you need to stabilize your new position. This question will stimulate you to find means of solidifying the new identity you have taken on for your new journey.

The question also stimulates you to reinforce your pursuit of the action steps to accomplish your goals. You are motivated to maintain continuous forward motion. At the same time, the process of stabilizing yourself will help you focus on enjoying the journey as opposed to thinking only of your destination. It opens up avenues for learning, personal development, and growth, which are all positive things you can gain from your transition journey.

An Evolving Line of Inquiry and Discovery That Is Uniquely Yours

This set of powerful questions is a framework for navigating all kinds of life transitions and career changes. They will provoke thoughts and evoke discovery on your part. Furthermore, they will elicit actions that will help you move forward.

I must emphasize that there are no solid lines demarcating these seven questions. There are no barriers indicating they cannot be crossed over. The questions are not a mathematical progression series that goes only in one direction. In fact, you may often have to go back and forth between the powerful questions in order to find the right answers in some instances.

Yes, you might start asking, "How do I get to that new place?" and still have to go back to the question, "Who am I in this present condition?" The whole process is an evolution. Some questions will evoke more discovery for you in certain life transitions than other questions. Even for people who are experiencing the same type of transitions, each particular individual's progression and sequence of finding answers will vary. No matter which sequence of questioning you take, the most important outcome is that you gain some form of awareness and are able to discover the necessary actions to get unstuck and move forward on a new smooth, paved road.

Just as you occupied the driver's position and took on leadership of your transition journey (see Chapter 8), you also need to take full ownership of the methods of search and discovery you employ in your navigation process. You decide the pace, the mix of powerful questions you use at each phase, and the methods of adapting your discovery to your own particular situation. When you do this, it will be easier for you to own your story, an essential element of finding meaning and significance in your experience.

An Avenue for Meaning and Significance

When you take ownership of your own story you will be willing to share it with others as described in Chapter 9. Furthermore, you will be stimulated to give back to others in your circles of influence and your community. Often this giving back has much to do with areas related to the transition you have been through.

Through this means of sharing, you are able to create a ripple effect, whereby the successes you have attained are multiplied in the lives of those you impact through your giving. This will enable you to discover even more meaning and enjoy a life of greater significance. Both Diane and Elena were able to find such meaning in their lives while impacting the lives of many other people in their communities.

Diane Spearheads the Launch of a New Foundation for Lupus

Diane has come a long way since that first moment her doctor informed her she had lupus. By shifting her mindset to one that affirmed the possibility of a new smooth, paved road in her future, she was able to see clearly and discover new options. She received help from her sister, who came to live with her for a while, as well as from a nurse and other forms of community support. She even found time to attend support group meetings for people with lupus.

All in all, Diane has found a new identity, and she continues to embrace and develop it. She has found a new way to run her business that is compatible with her current need to work fewer hours and take frequent breaks. In many respects, Diane feels stabilized on a new smooth, paved road.

However, Diane still feels a strong need to contribute in some way to discovering the cause of the disease she is suffering from. She knows about organizations in different parts of the world that are aimed at creating awareness about the disease and raising funds to support medical research for its cure. However, there is no such organization in Diane's country

Diane's desire to start such a local foundation for lupus is very strong. This project is a dream that Diane would not have thought of in normal circumstances. She has been in business for a long time and is quite an experienced entrepreneur; however, running a non-profit organization is not something that was on her radar before she was diagnosed with lupus.

As she initiates the project Diane knows this is a dream that is larger than her. However, the motivation to find a cure for lupus as well as increase the quality of life of people with the disease is a great force that keeps her going.

She researches her options for starting this new lupus foundation. One option she identifies is to create a social venture arm of her existing business. Diane takes this approach and obtains help to get it up and running. She always keeps in mind the fact that she should not exhaust herself working long hours.

Over the course of time Diane starts seeing the fruit of her efforts. The successes she achieves through the new foundation are a new source of fulfillment that Diane thrives upon on her new smooth, paved road.

Elena Volunteers Her Services for a Disaster Relief Organization

Elena, who relocated to Chicago after Hurricane Katrina, feels like she has laid her hands on a vital piece of information. When she hears that a delegation of Red

Cross volunteers are heading to a war-torn country for a three-month relief effort, Elena calls the telephone number indicated in the media story and requests more information. Somehow she feels instantly connected to the project.

She has never volunteered on such a project before. In fact, she is not the type of person who would typically take on humanitarian projects. Yes, she had loved working at her diner business in New Orleans, where she had had a chance to cater for many local people—a venture that is now history. And she has managed to keep up at her new job at the hotel restaurant, a job she has always considered temporary. She has indeed come a long way and has established new friendships in her Chicago neighborhood. But joining a relief effort is something altogether new, and she is amazed at how much she is drawn to the idea of participating in the project. Nevertheless, Elena decides to follow her heart and signs up as a volunteer. She does not exactly know the intricacies of the project, but she decides that should not be any hindrance to her involvement. After all, she has approached many aspects of her life in the past twenty-eight months just like that—like an act of faith.

Elena could not have been more thrilled when she begins working on the project. In fact, she discovers that her culinary skills are very much needed. She starts to think of this as her makeshift local diner again, where she helps to feed her fellow volunteers as well as some of the locals in the war-torn area.

As Elena shares her time and effort, she feels her life is more significant. Her life becomes more meaningful as she relates to the survivors of the disaster in concrete ways. While their experiences are not exactly the same as the one she went through, she feels a solid connection with this group of people. Through the power in that connection, she is able not only to give of herself, but also enjoy a sense of fulfillment.

The Way Forward

As you have progressed through this book, you have discovered the need to continue to decipher the way forward and to maintain continuous motion in that new direction. As you strive toward your new destination, remember that the journey is as important as reaching your goal. Take time to enjoy it.

Take forward the lessons you have learned and use them in future journeys you may embark upon. If you encounter any new detours, launch new lines of inquiry using the seven powerful questions. Acquire the sanity and strength you need to get unstuck from those detours and land back on a smooth, paved road.

With the right attitude and a positive mindset you will continue to multiply your wisdom and strength during any new transition you may experience. Do not neglect the important aspect of giving back to your community. As you share your experiences and knowledge you will continue to impact the lives of others in a positive way. And as you take on dreams larger than yourself you will find more meaning and enjoy a life of greater significance.

Take on the Power
of Your Uniqueness as You Go

As mentioned above, you are unique, and so is your process of acquiring the sanity and strength to overcome the challenges of change. The story that has been written during the whole process of going through your transition is uniquely yours and cannot be fabricated. The wealth of experiences you have had on the journey to your new destination are all part of this unique story. Any new obstacles on your new route or new delays in your journey will contribute to the richness of your experience.

As you recount your challenging moments, also recount the moments when you achieved victories over various issues. As you share your unique story you will multiply the sanity and strength you have acquired. You will increase your vitality by enabling others through the power of your story. And as you take ownership of your unique story, it will remain yours to keep and yours to add new chapters and sequels.

Keep on using the wisdom and power you have acquired in more areas of your life's journey.

Keep on multiplying the effect through sharing and caring.

Keep on impacting your community with the power of your experience.

Keep on enjoying your newly reignited passion for life!

Epilogue

Writing *Sanity and Strength* has been an interesting journey for me. When I first conceived the idea of the book, I was seeking to connect the wisdom for getting unstuck with the power to move on. Over time, that concept became threatened in many ways by a myriad of factors and influences in my personal and career lives.

However, the concept would just not go away, no matter the risks and hazards it faced. In fact, I experienced multiple entries onto, exits from, and reentries onto the pathway of putting the book together. During the periods of exit from the book project I was able to achieve some other important goals in my career life. However, those achievements felt limited because *Sanity and Strength* was still lurking in the womb of my mind, waiting to be born.

When I realized that this dream would not go away and, more importantly, that it seemed to be a fulcrum on which many other aspects of my career rested, I approached the situation by trying to get help to combine the various pieces I had managed to put together in my previous attempts to write the book. However, that approach did not work either. Having conceived *Sanity and Strength,* I was also meant to grow the concept, experience it as I put the various pieces together, then give birth to it.

I am so glad that this book is finally published. I am excited that the dream has been born. I am also thrilled that, along the way, I have acquired the wisdom for getting unstuck and the power for moving on in the complex situations surrounding my life.

I have found it fulfilling to have completed the book, and I will always cherish the experience of connecting the concepts of sanity and strength. The process of linking the two involved having to satisfy every prerequisite demanded by "sanity" alongside those required by "strength." It was similar to when I had to take basic science courses and score high grades in them before I could sign up for and pursue studies for my previous career in pharmacy.

I have immensely enjoyed the journey; the experience has been worth it. And I am glad to have the unique opportunity of sharing this book with you.

As you catch on to the theme of *Sanity and Strength* and acquire the wisdom to get unstuck and the power to move on from any complex transition you might be facing, I believe your success will also be multiplied and spread to far-reaching places.

Stay Connected and Engaged

Visit http://www.sanityandstrength.org to:

- Get more resources for navigating through life transitions and career changes

- Get the inside scoop on Sanity and Strength

- Read other Sanity and Strength stories

- Engage with a community of readers